Trauma and Orthopaedic Anaesthesia

Anaesthesia in a Nutshell

Geraldine Edge PhD FRCA
Consultant Anaesthetist
Royal National Orthopaedic Hospital
Stanmore, UK

Mary Fennelly FFARCSI MRCPI
Consultant Anaesthetist
Royal National Orthopaedic Hospital
Stanmore, UK

Series Editors: Neville Robinson and George Hall

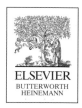

ELSEVIER
BUTTERWORTH
HEINEMANN

Edinburgh London New York Oxford Philadelphia St Louis Sydney Toronto 2004

ELSEVIER
BUTTERWORTH
HEINEMANN

First published 2004
    Reprinted 2006

ISBN 0 7506 5260 8

British Library Cataloguing in Publication Data
A catalogue record for this book is available from the British Library

Library of Congress Cataloguing in Publication Data
A catalogue record for this book is available from the Library of Congress

Notice
Medical knowledge is constantly changing. Standard safety precautions must be followed, but as new research and clinical experience broaden our knowledge, changes in treatment and drug therapy may become necessary or appropriate. Readers are advised to check the most current product information provided by the manufacturer of each drug to be administered to verify the recommended dose, the method and duration of administration, and contraindications. It is the responsibility of the practitioner, relying on experience and knowledge of the patient, to determine dosages and the best treatment for each individual patient. Neither the Publisher nor the author assumes any liability for any injury and/or damage to persons or property arising from this publication.

The Publisher

Printed in China

Contents

Series preface

Specialist registrars and senior house officers in anaesthesia are now trained by the use of modular educational programmes. In these short periods of intense training the anaesthetist must acquire a fundamental understanding of each anaesthetic speciality. To meet these needs, the trainee requires a concise, pocket-sized book that contains the core knowledge of each subject.

The aims of these 'nutshell' guides are two-fold: first, to provide trainees with the fundamental information necessary for the understanding and safe practice of anaesthesia in each speciality; and secondly, to cover all the key areas of the fellowship examination of the Royal College of Anaesthetists and so act as revision guides for trainees.

P. N. Robinson
G. M. Hall

Preface

Orthopaedic anaesthesia can be broadly seen to encompass all the different specialities of anaesthesia. Orthopaedic surgeons operate from the base of the skull to the end of the toe. In between, they perform elective and emergency surgery on both the thorax and pelvis. Anaesthesia is an exciting challenge and the anaesthetist encounters people at the extremes of health and age.

Many of the chapters complement each other and the book is by necessity written to avoid any unnecessary overlap in the text. This book is based on the practice that we use at the Royal National Hospital, Stanmore, and the book is written with the goal of assisting trainees at all stages of anaesthetic practice and for examination success.

Most anaesthetic trainees arrive at Stanmore expecting a period of unremitting joint replacement surgery and knee arthroscopies only to find that the majority of their paediatric training is about to take place and that any clinical problem that does not involve bone or metal requires 'anaesthetic' management!

We wish to thank Neville Robinson with the presentation of the text.

Geraldine Edge
Mary Fennelly

1

General Considerations for Orthopaedic Anaesthesia

Patients presenting for musculoskeletal surgery range from infants, with possible multiple congenital malformations, to the elderly with trauma, who have concurrent diseases, electrolyte disorders and are on a cocktail of different drugs. Interspersed throughout these age groups are adolescents who may present for scoliosis surgery, young adults with trauma for repair of joints, muscles and ligaments, and the elderly with the various forms of arthritis requiring elective joint replacement.

Nearly all anaesthetists in training or as consultants in general or specialist institutions are continually exposed to patients requiring elective orthopaedic or trauma surgery.

Box 1.1 shows the considerations that orthopaedic patients present when undergoing general or regional anaesthesia for surgery.

Patients present with incidental or concomitant disease. If disease is incidental then management should be directed to achieving optimisation of the medical condition. Only in major compound trauma necessitating immediate surgery can this simple rule be overlooked. Electrolyte abnormalities must be corrected prior to surgery in elderly patients. Concomitant disease is common in orthopaedic patients in specialist institutions. For example, scoliotic patients may have associated muscular dystrophies, and a full understanding of these diseases and their anaesthetic implications must be understood.

Drugs are important. Elderly patients often present taking aspirin for vascular disease and non-steroidal anti-inflammatory drugs for pain. These regimes often lead to gastric irritation, bleeding and subsequent anaemia, as well as renal damage and an anti-platelet effect. This may lead to increased haemorrhage and difficulty with surgical access, especially in spinal surgery, as well as having implications for the suitability of patients for epidural and other regional anaesthetic techniques. Additionally, thromboembolic prophylaxis in this group of patients becomes more complicated. There is no specific advice that can be

---

Box 1.1   General Considerations for Orthopaedic Anaesthesia

Age
Concomitant diseases
Drugs and interactions
Timing of surgery – elective or emergency
Higher incidence of latex allergy
Higher incidence of malignant hyperthermia
Haemorrhage
Analgesia
Antibiotic therapy and infection
Position of patient
Deep vein thrombosis and pulmonary embolism

---

offered for such patients – risk versus benefit analysis needs to be undertaken on each patient individually. Drugs such as clopidogrel and other anti-platelet medication need to be discontinued for at least 1 week prior to elective surgery.

Conditions of relevance to anaesthetists that should be sought for from patients include an increased propensity for malignant hyperthermia and latex allergy. The incidence of malignant hyperthermia is commonly cited as 1:10 000, but this is in the general hospital environment. The incidence is increased in males, children and young adults, in patients with congenital musculoskeletal disorders and, in particular, in patients with muscular dystrophies. Thus, if you work in a major orthopaedic hospital and undertake scoliosis anaesthesia in adolescents, you are more likely to encounter the problem. Latex allergy is more likely to be encountered in patients who have been exposed to multiple operations throughout their lives and who have been institutionalised. These people are often encountered in specialist orthopaedic hospitals.

Haemorrhage in orthopaedic surgery is notoriously difficult to estimate. In trauma and tumour surgery especially, the loss can be catastrophic and life threatening. Adequate preparation and careful replacement of blood and clotting factors is often needed. It is imperative to weigh swabs. In infants and small children, individual swabs should be weighed as they are discarded by the surgeon. Estimating blood loss can be confusing when large volumes of saline have been used to irrigate the surgical field.

Analgesia, whether pre- or postoperative, is an important consideration. Often, regional techniques are used to minimise postoperative discomfort and these are elucidated in the specific surgical chapters in this book. Routine systemic opiates and other drugs are also used. Following major spinal or limb surgery that may predispose to the compartment syndrome, epidural analgesia continued into the postoperative period may provide a 'gold standard' of pain relief but may also 'muddy the waters'. Ongoing assessment of the neurological status of the patient is mandatory if the sequelae of haematoma formation are to be avoided. Unless competent continuous neurological assessment is able to be undertaken, it is inappropriate to use regional techniques.

Infection and Antibiotic Therapy

Unlike bowel or gynaecological surgery, orthopaedic surgery is considered to be 'clean' in so far as there is no intrinsic source of bacteria. However, the incidence of infection after total hip replacement is reported as being 0.3–2.0% and is slightly higher after total knee replacement, being 0.6–4.0%. Infection after surgery involving prosthetic implants may be devastating. A postoperative infection prolongs hospital stay and the functional results of surgery are impaired. This may lead to the loss of prosthesis or limb amputation. Revision surgery is technically more difficult, time consuming and costly, and there is no guarantee that a second prosthesis may not also become infected. The prescription and administration of prophylactic antibiotics are primarily the responsibility of the surgeon. Nevertheless, the anaesthetist administers the majority of antibiotics.

Factors that increase the risk of infection include:

• Pre-existing systemic disease;
• The duration of surgery (excess of 3 hours);
• Superficial postoperative wound infection; and
• Previous arthroplasty of the same joint.

Available evidence does not justify additional per-operative doses of antibiotic for operations lasting less than 5 hours.

The infecting organisms are often of low virulence and usually originate from the patient's own skin. However, the skin of other operating staff, circulating dust particles and skin squames have also been implicated as sources of infection. Haematogenous spread from a distant infected focus or as a result of a bacteraemia-prone procedure may result in the late infection of a prosthesis that has been in situ for some time. Poor dental hygiene is often neglected as a source of infection.

General measures to reduce infection should be instituted prior to scheduling elective surgery and reversible patient risk factors should be corrected early. These include:

- Poor nutritional status (including obesity);
- Poor diabetic control; and
- Obvious skin infections.

Patients undergoing joint arthroplasty should undergo routine urinalysis some days before their operation, and it is worth noting that while proteinuria does not necessarily signify urinary tract infection, the presence of a urinary tract infection will invariably have associated proteinuria. Infection risk increases the longer the patient spends in hospital before an operation.

In the operating theatre, care must be taken to minimise release of bacteria and skin squames into the air. All hair should be covered, and facemasks serve to remind personnel that talking, coughing, and laughing over the incision are likely to contaminate the wound. The number of people in the theatre and their movement should be minimised, and unidirectorial laminar airflow is only of benefit if the turbulence caused by opening and closing doors is also minimised.

Surgical technique is fundamental to the prevention of wound infection. Antibiotic prophylaxis is no substitute for good antiseptic technique. Skin preparation must be adequate, with sufficient time allowed for alcoholic solutions to evaporate before the patient is draped. Haemostasis should be meticulous and the minimum time spent with the wound open.

Prophylactic antibiotics should only be used when there is a risk of infection occurring if they are not given. Box 1.2 illustrates the drugs and regimens commonly used for orthopaedic surgery. Although every regimen recommends more than one dose of antibiotic, there is no evidence that multiple-dose prophylaxis has any advantage over a single dose.

The likely source of infection of the bacteria needs to be identified; the activity of the chosen antibiotic needs to encompass the majority of the likely pathogens and the dose administered must provide effective tissue concentration prior to intraoperative bacterial contamination. For open fractures, early antibiotic administration and clinical vigilance are the keys to reducing infection. For elective surgery, antibiotics should be administered by intravenous injection 30–45 minutes prior to incision. The effective dose should be governed by the patient's weight and should be sufficient to maintain tissue levels above the minimum inhibitory concentration for 12 hours. Procedures

---

Box 1.2   Drug Regimens for Surgery

Primary and revisional joint surgery
  Intravenous cefuroxime three doses: 1.5 g on induction, 750 mg at 8
    and 16 hours post-induction (Remember, theoretically, a 10%
    crossover allergy exists between penicillin and the cephalosporins).
Infected joint surgery
  Regimens differ among patients depending on infecting organisms
  Intravenous teicoplanin 400 mg 12-hourly for three doses and
    24-hourly subsequently is used but must be drawn up according
    to instructions, with no bubbles as this decreases drug potency
    and concentration.
  Vancomycin
  Ciprocin

---

that last more than 5 hours or are associated with major blood loss
(1.5 l) or major intraoperative haemodilution may require a further dose
of antibiotics during the procedure. Peak bone concentrations occur
within 60 minutes of intravenous administration of most antibiotics
and, in practice, only the intravenous route guarantees predictable plasma and tissue concentrations at the start of surgery.

Systemic review by the NHS Research & Development Health
Technology Assessment has made the following recommendations.

- The choice of antibiotic is most usefully determined by local disease-
  specific information: usually a first- or second-generation cephalo-
  sporin or penicillinase-resistant penicillin is recommended.
- Vancomycin and teicoplanin are used if methicillin-resistant
  staphylococcus aureus is a problem on the unit or the patient is known
  to be colonised.
- If tissue samples are needed for microbiological assay, they should be
  taken early after incision and there is enough time to achieve high levels of antibiotic before the prosthesis is inserted.
- Blood-borne infection of implants may occur weeks or months after
  their introduction and patients should receive prompt treatment of any
  known infection elsewhere.
- Antibiotic cover should be given for bladder catheterisation in the
  perioperative period and, although there is no evidence that antibiotic
  cover is useful on catheter removal, the risk of urinary tract infection
  increases with the duration of catheterisation.

Box 1.3 shows the common infecting organisms and their frequency
after major joint replacement.

Box 1.3   Common Infecting Organisms and their Frequency after Major Joint Replacement

Coagulase negative staphylococcus	25–45%
Staphylococcus aureus	19–25%
Polymicrobial	3–16%
Anaerobic Gram-negative bacilli	7–13%
Streptococci	2–11%
Anaerobes	6–9%
Enterococci	3–5%
Diptheroids	2–5%

Bacteraemia during dental treatment is common and some surgeons recommend prophylaxis for the first 3 months following joint replacement surgery when the risk of haematogenous spread is highest.

Positioning

Optimal positioning that allows adequate surgical access is crucial for successful surgery. It is important that physiological changes are lessened. Priorities include:

- Adequate surgical exposure;
- Minimal blood loss; and
- Avoidance of nerve injuries or pressure sores.

Positioning the patient requires the close cooperation of all the members of the theatre team. The salient problems associated with the supine, prone, lateral decubitus and sitting positions will be discussed, as well as the management of the patient on the fracture table. Box 1.4 summarises these problems.

Supine Position

The supine position is essentially devoid of major cardiovascular consequences and the main problems arise from nerve compression. The nerves most vulnerable to injury are those of the upper extremities, specifically the brachial plexus and the ulnar nerves. Brachial plexus injuries can occur with excessive head rotation and neck hyperextension (as in shoulder surgery). Any traction from pulling the patient can lead to brachial plexus damage.

When the arm is positioned with the palm pronated or abducted on an arm board, the ulnar nerve is exposed and vulnerable to compression. It is essential to pad the elbow and limit abduction to 90 degrees to

---

Box 1.4   Major Problems Associated with Positioning Patients

---

Supine
  Brachial plexus and ulnar nerve injuries
Prone
  Decreased venous return
  Increased work of breathing
  Tracheal tube removal or disconnection
  Secure venous cannulae
  Nerve compression
  Ocular pressure
  Potential for compartment syndrome
Lateral decubitus
  Pressure effects
  Nerve injuries
  Corneal abrasions
  Respiratory imbalance
  Monitoring equipment
Sitting
  Cardiovascular instability
  Air embolism
  Quadriplegia

---

lessen this problem. Orthopaedic surgery in the modified lithotomy position can cause sciatic and common peroneal nerve compression. The incidence and severity of nerve damage increases with the duration of the surgery.

Prone Position

The prone position is most commonly used in spinal surgery but is also used for surgery on the back of the leg and often in tendo-achilles repair. It is essential when positioning patients in the prone position that there is adequate thoracic and pelvic support so that the anterior abdominal wall hangs freely – this minimises the major haemodynamic and respiratory effects. Pressure on the abdominal wall increases pressure within the abdominal wall cavity and compresses the inferior vena caval and femoral veins and, as a result, venous return can be compromised. Cardiac output and blood pressure decrease. Venous return to the heart is facilitated by alternative routes, especially via the vertebral venous plexus, which will become distended and interfere with surgical access and cause haemorrhage! The diaphragm may also be pushed upwards by abdominal wall compression and this increases the work of breathing and alters ventilation/perfusion ratios in the lung. Positive-pressure ventilation can actually improve oxygenation in the prone position.

The tracheal tube must be secured and positioned carefully. Accidental removal from the trachea is catastrophic in the prone position. Kinking of the tube is normally avoided by insertion of an armour-reinforced tube. All lines must be securely strapped.

Nerve compression must be avoided in the prone position. Positioning the head correctly is crucial and it should be maintained in a neutral position with the weight distributed evenly to the forehead, maxilla and mandible. The eyes should be taped closed and then padded, and no pressure should be exerted over them. Any compression of the eyes, even for a short time, can cause optic nerve ischaemia or central retinal artery thrombosis. The head and neck should be checked throughout surgery. Vigorous surgical techniques such as stripping muscles off the vertebrae with the Cobb elevator can cause significant head and neck movement and displacement of any previously meticulously sited facial support. The brachial plexus is vulnerable throughout its entire length in the prone position and stretch injuries are common. Other nerves that must be protected include the ulnar at the elbow and the median at the wrist. Ulnar nerve injury is more common after general anaesthesia than neural blockade. The femoral nerve may be compressed and skin necrosis of the feet has been reported from prolonged pressure.

Care must be taken to avoid compromising the arterial supply and venous drainage of the lower limbs to preclude muscle ischaemia and the compartment syndrome. Sharp angulation of the hips or knees can severely restrict circulation of the lower limbs and must be avoided. A good rule of thumb is to avoid extension or flexion of joints of more than 90 degrees, if possible.

A variety of frames, mattresses (commonly the Montreal mattress) and ream rolls are available, and a variety of padded arm boards are available to prevent upper limb nerve compression for these patients. However, differently shaped patients require differing types of supports, and imaginative intervention may be required.

Lateral Position

The lateral position is often used for hip surgery and for the anterior approach to the spine. Positioning is facilitated by deflatable bean-bags or a series of chest and pelvic supports. Careful attention to the elbows and the wrists will ensure that nerve injuries of the upper limbs do not occur. Careful padding of vulnerable areas is mandatory.

The consequences of perfusion mismatch can be reduced by the application of positive end-expiratory pressure if the patient's lungs are ventilated. If the dependent limbs are compressed in the initial positioning of the patient then the patency of indwelling urinary, arterial and central venous catheters is affected. The noninvasive blood pressure cuff functions improperly if compressed when on the lower limb and is normally placed on the upper arm. Corneal abrasions can occur if the dependent eye is accidentally open and scratched by the pillow. Tape the eyes shut but ensure that the eye lashes are not folded into the conjunctiva.

Sitting Position

The sitting position offers easy surgical access for cervical spine surgery and provides better venous and cerebrospinal fluid drainage. Cardiovascular compromise occurs in this position, especially in elderly patients. The main risks include venous air embolism (thus, end-tidal carbon dioxide must be checked with vigilance) and quadriplegia. This rare complication is an indication for ongoing spinal cord monitoring. Quadriplegia may be due to stretching of the cord or inadequate cord perfusion in this position. Patients with proven cervical stenosis should never be operated on in this position because of this risk. Although the sitting position is increasingly rare for neurosurgery, for the occasional patient with ankylosing spondylitis, this position is unavoidable.

Orthopaedic Table

The fracture or traction table is specifically designed to facilitate access to the lower limbs in order to pin lower extremity and pelvic fractures. The upper limbs and body are supported while the limbs are suspended in boots. Pressure points must be padded to avoid nerve compression. Be aware that the patient can be pulled from the original position during vigorous surgery and accidental tracheal disconnection has been described. A post is placed between the legs to stop movement, and excessive pressure here can cause a loss of perineal sensation. Medicolegally, this is an expensive complication.

Deep Vein Thrombosis and Thromboembolic Prophylaxis

Deep vein thrombosis (DVT) is the commonest cause of readmission to hospital after joint replacement surgery, contributing to postoperative morbidity and mortality, and is a significant cause of delayed discharge home. Venous thromboembolism does occur spontaneously in people who are ambulant, and in 50% of these individuals no predisposing factor can be identified. In the remaining 50% of this 'normal' group, associated risk factors may include:

- Malignant disease;
- Thrombophilia;
- Oral contraceptive medication; and
- Varicose veins or previous thrombosis.

Age is a definite risk factor and risk rises linearly after the age of 50 years.

Estimates of the incidence of venous thrombosis after hip fracture range from 15% to 48%; after elective total knee replacement from 40–80% and after total hip replacement from 40–70%. In 9–20% of this latter group of patients, the thrombus develops in the deep veins of the thigh and has a greater potential to embolise to the lungs. Of patients who develop proximal deep vein thrombosis, 5–10% will develop a pulmonary embolus and approximately 10% of pulmonary emboli are fatal.

Most studies of the prevalence of pulmonary embolism are based on sudden death in 'at-risk' groups of patients. Many of these studies do not have post-mortem confirmation of pulmonary embolus. With this in mind, published data provide the following information for death due to:

- Pulmonary embolus following emergency surgery for fractured neck of femur, 4–7%;
- Elective hip replacement, 0.3–1.7%; and
- Elective general surgery, 0.1–0.8%.

The long-term sequelae of DVT are poorly elucidated but up to one-third of patients experience post-thrombolic problems or post-phlebitic syndrome within 5–10 years.

Abnormalities of flow or stasis occur after prolonged immobility or confinement to bed. With all surgical approaches to the hip, dislocation of the femoral head kinks the femoral vein and it is not until reduction of the head of the femur into the acetabulum that venous flow is re-established during hip arthroplasty.

The risk factors for deep vein thrombosis are shown in Box 1.5.

Thrombosis, after surgery, is difficult to diagnose – pain, swelling, tenderness and erythema of the lower limb accompany surgery, and thrombosis in the thigh is often clinically silent. Specific clinical features include:

- Tenderness along the entire deep vein system;
- Swelling of the entire leg with more than 3 cm difference in calf circumference;

- Pitting oedema; and
- Dilation of superficial veins.

The diagnosis is normally confirmed by Doppler ultrasonography.

The prevention of DVT and the use antithrombotic prophylaxis are based upon the risk factors shown in Box 1.6.

Spinal and epidural anaesthesia reduce the risk of DVT by 20%. It is not known whether their effect is additive with other methods.

Box 1.5   Risk Factors for Deep Vein Thrombosis (DVT)

Past history of venous thromboembolism.
Prolonged immobility – confinement to bed and lower limb paralysis.
Oestrogen therapy – to fully reverse the prothrombotic effects of oestrogen oral contraceptives, treatment should be discontinued for 6 weeks prior to any elective surgery. The risk of DVT associated with continued oestrogen contraception (50:100 000) has to be balanced against the slightly increased risk of DVT associated with pregnancy (60:100 000). Progesterone-only oral contraceptive medication carries no increased risk of DVT formation. With postmenopausal hormone replacement therapy (HRT), the risk of DVT is approximately half that of oestrogen oral contraception, but patients are generally less willing to discontinue treatment. There is no published information on the specific effects of continued HRT and it is therefore perceived as safe.
Hypercoagulable states – inherited (protein C and protein S deficiency, antithrombin deficiency, activated protein C resistance) and acquired (myeloproliferative disease, polycythaemia, antiphospholipid antibodies in systemic lupus erythromatosus).
Malignant disease – especially adenocarcinoma.

Box 1.6   Risk Factors for Thrombosis after Surgery

Low risk
   Minor surgery <30 minutes duration – no other risk factors
Medium risk
   a)   Major surgery >40 years old with other risk factors present
   b)   Minor surgery, trauma or illness with a past history of venous thromboembolism
High risk
   a)   Major orthopaedic surgery, fractured hip, pelvis or knee
   b)   Abdominal or pelvic surgery for cancer
   c)   Major surgery in a patient with a past medical history of venous thromboembolism
   d)   Lower limb paralysis or amputation

DVT prophylaxis employs both mechanical and pharmacological strategies.

Mechanical Methods

The mechanical methods include graduated compression stockings, which must be fitted meticulously, to increase the flow of blood in leg veins. Although they have been shown to be more effective in general surgery than arthroplasty, nevertheless, there is a significant reduction in the rate of DVT after hip and knee arthroplasty when they are used. Their use is contraindicated where there is existing oedema or ulceration of the leg. Foot pumps and other compressive devices work by intermittent inflation of a pneumatic device located in a bootee. They are expensive, noisy and generally disliked by patients. Bootees with an inflatable sole are as effective as those enclosing the entire calf. They have been shown to be effective in the prevention of subclinical thrombosis and some trials have suggested that they are as efficacious as low molecular weight heparin (LMWH).

Pharmacological Method

The pharmacological method consists of the use of LMWH started subcutaneously 12 hours preoperatively and generally used daily for 5 days postoperatively or until the risk factors are minimal. Unfractionated heparin is now used only in the initial treatment of DVT, either by intravenous infusion or subcutaneous injection. The contraindications to LMWH therapy include:

- Bleeding diathesis;
- Active peptic ulcer disease;
- Recent head injury or stroke; and
- Known drug hypersensitivity.

Aspirin alters platelet aggregation but has not been found to be reliably effective in preventing DVT after hip and knee surgery. Designer drugs are being developed in response to continuing mortality and morbidity from DVT despite existing management protocols. Fondaparinux sodium is a synthetic drug and differs from LMWH in both pharmacokinetics and clinical efficacy. Early trials report that this drug has a similar safety profile to LMWH enoxaparin but produced a 50% greater reduction in thromboembolic events. Watch this space!

For patients in the low-risk category, no more prophylaxis is recommended than early mobilisation. For medium-risk patients, recommendations are for graduated compression stockings, intermittent pneumatic compression or daily LMWH. For high-risk patients, stockings, compression devices and LMWH are all recommended. For patients deemed to be at very great risk, prolonged anticoagulation may be instituted.

The management of a proven DVT consists of starting warfarin in conjunction with heparin or LMWH. Administration should be concomitant for 5 days and until INR >2. Daily platelet counts are required when heparin is used. Heparin and warfarin prevent extension of the thrombus and embolisation.

The clinical features of pulmonary embolism are neither sensitive nor specific. Dyspnoea is the most frequent symptom, occurring in 75% of patients, with pleuritic chest pain occurring in 50%. Haemoptysis occurs after 24 hours as the result of infarcted lung tissue and is seen in fewer than 25% of patients. An infiltrate is seen on the chest X-ray in approximately 50% of patients at the time of onset. The absence of a positive diagnosis for DVT does not exclude the possibility of an acute pulmonary embolus. Pulmonary embolism may present with collapse, shock and cardiac arrest.

The diagnosis is confirmed by the use of a ventilation–perfusion (V/Q) lung scan. A normal lung scan excludes an embolus but an abnormal scan does not confirm an embolus. This investigation is diagnostic in 30% of cases. The 'classic' electrocardiogram changes of 'S1, Q3, T3' are rarely seen. More commonly, there is right axis deviation, right bundle branch block and T inversion in leads V1–4. Spiral computed tomography scanning is more reliable than V/Q scanning but is limited to the detection of emboli in large vessels.

Supportive treatment and anticoagulation are the mainstay of treatment of suspected or confirmed pulmonary embolus. Oxygen administration and circulatory support are instituted as required. As with the treatment of DVT, heparin and warfarin are started as soon as possible and given concomitantly for 5 days. Pulmonary embolectomy should theoretically be carried out if the occlusion is greater than 75%; in practice, the small group of patients who may benefit from this procedure rarely survive long enough to reach the operating theatre. Vena caval filters are indicated when recurrent pulmonary emboli occur or there is confirmed thrombus in the deep veins above the thigh in a high-risk surgical patient. With this device in situ, the incidence of clinically proven embolus is under 3% when used in conjunction with anticoagulation.

The use of regional and, in particular, epidural anaesthesia in patients receiving LMWH is controversial. The incidence of epidural haematoma in the UK is 1:200 000, which is rare but nevertheless catastrophic when it occurs. Current practice includes individual risk/benefit analysis, but safe practice allows for an epidural catheter to be inserted 8–12 hours after a dose of LMWH and for the catheter to be removed 6 hours after a dose. By following this rule, the risk is further minimised.

2

Specific Considerations for Orthopaedic Anaesthesia

Orthopaedic surgery is associated with several conditions and complications of which the anaesthetist must be aware.

Compartment Syndrome

Compartment syndrome is defined as the elevation of tissue pressure above vascular perfusion pressure resulting in ischaemia of the tissues within an anatomical muscle compartment. It can develop in any part of the body when the pressure increases inside an inelastic boundary. Such inelastic boundaries, comprising layers of fascia and periosteum, surround skeletal muscle and thus the four compartments of the forearm and lower leg are most at risk. However, the syndrome may also develop in the hand, foot, upper arm, thigh and buttock. The build-up of pressure within the tissue may result from either:

- A decrease in compartment size, e.g. tight bandages or plaster of Paris; or
- From an increase of volume within the compartment, e.g. bleeding, oedema or increases in capillary pressure due to exercise or venous obstruction.

As the boundaries of the compartment are noncompliant, pressure increases cannot dissipate. Eventually, the rise in pressure exceeds perfusion pressure, resulting in acute muscle ischaemia and then necrosis. In the long term, this will eventually result in limb paralysis and contracture. The best-known example of this condition is Volkmann's ischaemic contracture.

The classic signs of compartment syndrome are said to be pain, parasthesia, pallor and pulselessness, although the only consistent symptoms are pain and parasthesia. By the time pallor and pulselessness have occurred, ischaemia is irreversible. Indeed, pulselessness is extremely unreliable as a sign; peripheral pulses are palpable unless major arterial injury has occurred. Tissues in the affected limb will appear distended and are tense on palpation. Pain is the earliest and most reliable symptom in compartment syndrome, particularly pain that is out of proportion to the injury. However, many of these patients have painful injuries, e.g. fracture or crush injuries, and whether pain is disproportional is a subjective assessment. More importantly, increasing pain, or increasing requirement for analgesia after a period of well-controlled pain, should always carry a high index of suspicion.

The pain is described as a deep sensation of unrelenting pressure that may be throbbing in character. Parasthesia may eventually progress to hyperaesthesia or anaesthesia. Passive extension of fingers or toes will exacerbate the pain. Sensory changes usually precede motor changes. Early parasthesia may be confined to the dermatome supplied by the nerves passing through the affected compartment. By the time paralysis has occurred, ischaemic damage will be irreversible.

Measurement of intracompartmental tissue pressure is a valuable means of making a definitive diagnosis. Although special kits are commercially available, a wide-bore cannula, fixed to a standard arterial pressure transducer and introduced into the compartment, provides a quick and accurate bedside test. Tissue pressures in the supine lower leg range between 9 and 15 mmHg normally. Ischaemia is inevitable at pressures above 50 mmHg but may start as low as 30 mmHg. The duration of elevated intracompartmental pressure is directly related to the resulting tissue damage.

If compartment syndrome is suspected, all circumferential dressings must be removed and plaster casts must be split to skin along the entire length immediately. A tissue pressure of 30 mmHg is an indication for urgent surgical decompression. Ischaemic muscle, which will appear brownish and noncontractile, requires excision. The fascia is left open and as muscle bulges through the wound, skin closure may not be possible. Intravenous fluid regimens must compensate for fluid lost from large raw areas.

Although compartment syndrome is a recognised complication of limb surgery, it is also occasionally a complication of surgical positioning where acute joint flexion causes localised pressure that may obstruct the venous return from a limb. It has also been reported as a result of prolonged muscle stimulation from spinal cord monitoring during spinal surgery. Eliciting a complaint suggestive of compartment syndrome therefore often falls to the anaesthetist, who is usually the first doctor to speak to the patient after surgery. It cannot be overemphasised that the onset of compartment syndrome is heralded by pain, and breakthrough pain in the light of previously adequate, especially epidural, analgesia may be pathognomonic.

Cast Syndrome

Cast syndrome is also known as the 'superior mesenteric artery syndrome' and occurs when gastric outflow is obstructed by occlusion of the third part of the duodenum. The third part of the duodenum passes between the superior mesenteric artery anteriorly and the aorta and vertebral column posteriorly. When the angle between the superior mesenteric artery and aorta is narrowed, the duodenum becomes compressed and obstructed.

Cast syndrome has been reported in patients with scoliosis, multiple trauma, burns and following application of plaster jackets or plaster body spicas. In scoliosis, it occurs following correction of the curve by surgical instrumentation or application of a cast after traction has been applied. Correction of the curve of the spine narrows the angle between the superior mesenteric artery and aorta, thereby occluding the lumen of the duodenum and causing high intestinal obstruction.

The syndrome presents with nausea and vomiting. Asymptomatic intervals occur between episodes of vomiting, which decompresses the stomach. Abdominal distension is variable but the lower abdomen remains soft with active bowel sounds. Distension of the stomach increases downward pressure on the duodenum and aggravates the obstruction.

The diagnosis requires a high level of suspicion, particularly as nausea and vomiting is likely to be attributed to the anaesthetic and analgesia during the postoperative period. Plain abdominal X-ray will usually confirm the diagnosis, with the film showing a distended stomach and little gas in the lower bowel. Gastrografin swallow demonstrates dilation of the proximal duodenum, obstruction of the third part of the duodenum and delayed gastric emptying. Later films will differentiate between partial and complete obstruction.

Prolonged vomiting will cause dehydration and electrolyte imbalance, and intravenous rehydration and nutrition should be started early. Oral intake should be restricted and the stomach decompressed by nasogastric suctioning. Nursing the patient in a left lateral, head-down position encourages relief of the obstruction.

Cast syndrome usually resolves within 48–72 hours. When due to the application of a cast or spica, removal may be necessary if vomiting has not resolved within 72 hours. Rarely, surgical intervention may be required with side-to-side duodenojejunostomy being the procedure of choice. Deaths have been reported in the untreated syndrome.

Tourniquets

Tourniquets are used to provide a bloodless field for surgery on the extremities and are applied after exsanguination of the limb. This may be achieved by applying a rubber bandage under tension, starting distally and working proximally (the method of choice for hands and feet in adults or the entire limb in small children). In adults, a 'rubber sausage' (more correctly called a Rhys-Davies exsanguinator) is applied prior to tourniquet inflation. Where tissues are friable or infection or tumours are present, simple elevation for 2 minutes (by the clock) is usually effective. Simple elevation is also preferable when deep vein thrombosis is suspected.

The majority of tourniquets in everyday use are pneumatic, i.e. inflatable. An integrated, accurate pressure gauge adds an element of safety. An automatic device that inflates rapidly to a pre-set pressure which is constantly regulated is ideal but inflation with a hand pump is satisfactory. Anaeroid gauges require frequent calibration checks. Although this is easily and accurately achieved using a mercury manometer, this is rarely carried out. Errors in calibration have been found to be over 100%!

Lengths of rubber tubing tied or clipped around the base of digits are commonly used; the pressure applied is unknown and, provided their application is of short duration, these ad hoc systems do not appear to cause great problems.

Pneumatic tourniquets are available in a huge range of lengths and widths, but most operating theatres stock only a few (and never of a size to suit the surgeon!). The width for an adult arm should be at least 10 cm, with wider cuffs available for obese patients. Cuffs for the leg should be curved so as to conform to conical thighs; this allows more uniform dissipation of pressure. It should be noted that wide tourniquet cuffs are more effective at lower pressures than are narrow ones. Considerations for tourniquets are shown in Box 2.1.

There is little agreement about inflation pressures for tourniquets although, in general, greater pressures than necessary are usually used. The correct pressure will depend on the blood pressure and diameter of the limb. For the upper limb, pressures of 135–255 mmHg achieve satisfactory arterial occlusion. Corresponding pressures in the lower limb range from 175 to 300 mmHg. If the pneumatic cuff leaks and inflating pressures fall below systolic pressure, the veins will become engorged and bleeding will be torrential. If the cuff cannot be exchanged, it must be removed entirely and surgery proceed without tourniquet.

There is no absolute rule as to how long a tourniquet cuff may remain inflated. The safe period will vary with the age of the patient and the blood supply to the limb. Nerve paralysis may result from excessive pressure or excessive duration of application. If the operation takes more than 2 hours, it is probably safest to abandon the tourniquet after

---

Box 2.1   Considerations for Tourniquets

Type of tourniquet
Size
Pressure
   Arm – systolic + 50 mmHg
   Leg – systolic + 100 mmHg
   Obese limbs – twice systolic pressure
Time – in fit healthy adults
   1 hour – safe
   1.5 hours – maximum
   2 hours – release tourniquet
Nerve damage
Skin damage
Site
Note keeping

---

this time. Deflation of the tourniquet for 5 minutes and then reinflation does not protect the nerve from damage. Nerve paralysis is the result of direct pressure. The duration of inflation of the tourniquet cuff should be moderated in:

- The elderly;
- Patients on steroids; and
- Patients who are alcoholic, diabetic or have other neuropathies.

Pneumatic cuffs should only be placed around the upper arm or upper thigh. They should not be used around the forearm, calf, wrist or ankle.

It has been estimated that a major complication directly attributable to tourniquet use occurs in 1:8000 patients. Fragile skin may be damaged in patients with rheumatoid arthritis, Ehlers-Danlos syndrome, epidermolysis bullosa or on high-dose steroids. Exsanguination may lead to dissemination of infection, tumour or mobilisation of a deep vein thrombosis. Calcified blood vessels may be incompressible. Irritant skin preparation solutions under the cuff may cause maceration or, when diathermy is used, burns.

The use of tourniquets in patients with sickle cell disease is contentious. Use in patients with sickle cell trait is acceptable providing exsanguination is scrupulous. Sickle cell crises may occur in homozygous patients, and tourniquets should not be used.

Site and type of cuff, method of exsanguination, the cuff pressure and duration of application should all be noted. Return of circulation should be noted and postoperative application of the pulse oximeter to the digits can be reassuring for both the surgeon and the anaesthetist.

Methyl Methacrylate Cement

A number of prosthetic devices require fixation using the acrylic polymer methyl methacrylate. This is presented as a liquid monomer which, when mixed in solution, becomes a solid polymer. When inserted into a bone, an expanding exothermic interface is created between the bone and the prosthesis. This, in an unvented bone, can lead to an increase in the intramedullary pressure of the bone, with the resultant 'syndrome' of hypotension, hypoxaemia, dysrhythmias, and even cardiac arrest occurring.

It is not fully understood why this happens. Most probably, it is due to embolism from the contents of the shaft of the bone (air, fat, stem cells and endothelial cells), but it also may be due to allergy or the exothermic nature of the chemical reaction. There is less cardiovascular instability if the blood volume is normal and, therefore, meticulous volume replacement should occur during joint surgery. Many anaesthetists 'lighten' anaesthesia slightly prior to cement insertion, and all are vigilant (often giving 100% oxygen) to maintain the oxygen saturation if hypoxaemia occurs. Surgeons must be persuaded that preventing increases in the medullary pressure by venting the canal or by inserting the cement into the distal part of the bone first is a useful intervention.

These ventilation/perfusion mismatch changes are usually brief, and this has been attributed to the small size of the embolic particles. If a tourniquet has been used, embolised particles will be retained within the venous circulation and haemodynamic instability will be delayed until the tourniquet is released.

The larger the volume of cement used (beware of the surgical request for two or three mixes), the more profound the systemic effects can be. Many anaesthetists habitually draw up adrenaline when surgery for massive prosthetic replacement is undertaken. This is particularly important when proximal femoral replacement is performed.

Fat Embolism

Fat embolism is defined as the presence of fat droplets in lung parenchyma and peripheral microcirculation following trauma. It is particularly associated with fractures of long bones, and fat droplets may be demonstrated in up to 90% of these patients. Fat emboli have also been demonstrated after prosthetic joint replacement, bone marrow transplant, acute pancreatitis and external cardiac massage.

Fat embolism syndrome (FES) comprises signs affecting the lungs, central nervous system and skin and is due to the presence of fat droplets in the microcirculation. The majority of patients with fat emboli are asymptomatic. Isolated respiratory compromise occurs in 30% of patients with fat droplets in the blood but only 1–5% develop the full triad of signs. The onset of the syndrome usually occurs 2–3 days after injury but may occur as early as 12 hours after injury.

A long bone fracture causes disruption of fat cells within the bone marrow and the release of small fat globules into the circulation via torn venules in the marrow cavity. These small fat globules become coated with platelets, which release several biochemical mediators that produce local vasospasm and bronchospasm with ventilation/perfusion mismatch and capillary congestion. It is unlikely that vascular occlusion alone is the cause of the severe pulmonary and neurological problems that occur in FES. It has been suggested that hypoxia and hypoperfusion cause cellular disruption and the release of tissue lipases, which hydrolyse fat within emboli, increasing fatty acids and glycerol concentration. In pulmonary capillaries, this causes vesiculation and disruption of the basement membrane.

Fat emboli from bone marrow enter the venous circulation to reach the lungs. Central nervous system and skin manifestations suggest that the emboli have gained access to the arterial side of the circulation either by passage through alveolar capillaries or via precapillary shunts that have opened in response to raised pulmonary pressure. The neurological features of FES are due to the same biochemical and histological changes that occur in the lungs.

The main features of fat embolism syndrome are shown in Box 2.2.

Box 2.2   Features of Fat Embolism

Major
  Respiratory insufficiency – 75%
  Cerebral manifestations – 86%
  Petechial rash – 60%
Minor
  Pyrexia
  Tachycardia
  Retinal signs
  Renal manifestations
  Jaundice
  Fat macroglobulinaemia

The clinical diagnosis rests on the presence of one major and four minor signs or on the basis of respiratory criteria alone in a patient with a long bone fracture. These criteria are a $PaO_2 < 8$ kPa, $PaCO_2 > 7.5$ kPa or a pH < 7.3 and tachypnoea >35/min.

Hypoxaemia precedes the onset of dyspnoea and tachypnoea. Examination reveals fine inspiratory crackles and, histologically, fat globules may be seen in the sputum. Blood gas abnormalities precede X-ray changes by several hours but a later chest X-ray will reveal bilateral fluffy shadows. Ten per cent of patients develop respiratory failure with features of acute respiratory distress syndrome.

Central nervous system involvement presents as an encephalopathy 6–12 hours before respiratory signs but it is rare for a patient to have neurological signs without respiratory involvement. Clinically, the patient develops an acute confusional state that does not improve on administration of oxygen (although hypoxia will cause exacerbation). A small number of patients develop a decreased level of consciousness with focal signs including aphasia, apraxia, hemiplegia and anisocoria.

Skin signs present as a petechial rash within 36 hours of injury that is most readily seen in the conjunctiva and mucous membranes in the mouth. The rash is confined to the upper trunk, particularly the neck and the axillae. It is self-limiting and usually disappears within 1 week.

A large number of specific treatments have been tried but none has been shown to be of benefit. These include alcohol, heparin, aprotinin and steroids. The mainstay of treatment is respiratory support and, in the majority of cases, recovery occurs spontaneously and completely. Early fixation of fractures has been shown to reduce the incidence of fat embolism syndrome and hypovolaemia has been shown to increase susceptibility to the development of the syndrome. The role of steroids is controversial but they are generally considered to be detrimental after the first 24 hours. Heparin therapy has not been demonstrated to be effective.

As FES is due to trauma, it is difficult to assess any sequelae due to the syndrome per se. The risk of death is 5–15% and is directly related to the severity of respiratory insufficiency. Long-term morbidity is related to the development of focal neurological deficits but the prognosis is usually good and full recovery should be expected.

Latex Allergy

Although latex allergy is not a condition specific to patients presenting for orthopaedic surgery, it is the group of patients in which it occurs most frequently, particularly in those who require multiple procedures throughout their lives. Latex is the white milky liquid produced by the rubber tree *Hevea brasiliensis* and is the raw material from which rubber is made. Rubber-based items are ubiquitous in medicine, not just in gloves but in dressings, mattress covers and tubing connectors, as well as seals on vials and ampoules.

The route of sensitisation (skin, mucosa or intravascular), the source of protein (glove, catheter, endotracheal tube, etc.), the type of latex (high or low ammoniated) and individual immune response (atopy) may result in variations in the severity of the reaction. Starch powder in gloves absorbs and binds protein readily and may have a role in making the antigens airborne.

The manifestations of anaphylactic reaction range from the mildly inconvenient (rhinitis, urticaria) through to those which are life threatening (cardiovascular collapse, angioedema, bronchoconstriction) and death. The clinical signs are shown in Box 2.3. Latex allergy should be considered as the main cause of delayed intraoperative anaphylaxis during surgery. It often appears 30–45 minutes into surgery.

Between 3% and 15% of people who wear surgical gloves during the course of their daily work become sensitised to latex. In the general population, the prevalence of latex sensitivity is 1:1000 although 4% of atopic individuals are latex sensitive. The risk of developing an allergy is generally higher in females and certain specific patient groups have been shown to have high rates of latex allergy. These groups are shown to include the following.

1. Spina bifida: the reported prevalence of latex allergy ranges from 18% to 68% in this group. This may be related to exposure during early surgery and subsequent multiple urinary tract instrumentation procedures. In general, all patients with spina bifida, even those who give no history of hypersensitivity, should be treated as though they are latex sensitive.

Box 2.3   Clinical Signs of Latex Allergy

Cutaneous manifestations: pruritis, erythema, non-urticaria rash, urticaria – local or generalised
Mucosal manifestations: oedema, angioedema, rhinitis, conjunctivitis
Respiratory tract: cough, dyspnoea, asthma, bronchospasm, stridor
Systemic reactions: hypotension due to increased vascular permeability, disseminated intravascular coagulation, myocardial depression, death

2. Patients with genitourinary tract anomalies.
3. Atopic patients with previous history of eczema and allergic asthma. Theoretically, patients with allergies to certain fruit (bananas, avocados, chestnuts and kiwi fruit) may also be more prone to developing latex allergy. This is because in vitro testing has shown that latex and these fruit share some common antigens. However, as yet, there is no epidemiological evidence to support any clinical concerns.
4. Patients who have undergone multiple general surgical procedures, e.g. patients with chronic spinal injury.

Latex allergy is not confined to these groups and the condition is sufficiently rare that specific questions designed to elicit a history of allergy to latex or rubber articles are rarely asked during the preoperative visit. If a history consistent with latex allergy is obtained, elective surgery should be deferred until the diagnosis can be confirmed or excluded.

Latex sensitivity can be confirmed by in vivo, ex vivo, and in vitro testing. Specificity will depend on the antigen preparation used and pure latex solution is rarely available. Skin prick testing is one of the most useful tests and a positive wheal and flare response is diagnostic. A negative response does not absolutely exclude the diagnosis of latex allergy. The procedure may induce a systemic anaphylactic reaction in acutely sensitive individuals and should only be undertaken by experienced clinicians with resuscitation facilities available. RAST (radio allegro sorbent testing) is designed to detect the presence of circulating IgE antibodies to latex antigen. It is less reliable and therefore less useful than skin prick testing and concordance between the two techniques is lacking. Basophil histamine release provides accurate results in experienced hands but is generally less readily available. Provocation testing relies on eliciting a reaction following controlled exposure to the antigen. Results are diagnostic but the procedure exposes the patient to the risk of a significant reaction.

The management of a patient with clear evidence of latex sensitivity requires the provision of a latex-free environment, both in the operating theatre and on the ward. In some hospitals, manufacturers of all equipment are contacted using a standard letter requesting details of the latex or rubber content in each product. This provides a database that can be regularly updated and recommendations can be made for the purchase of latex-free substitutes. The problem and consequences of latex allergy are now sufficiently well known for manufacturers to be actively seeking alternatives to latex components.

Some hospitals favour the provision of a 'latex-free' trolley where all the items are known to be latex free, e.g. syringes, intravenous administration sets, tracheal tubing and urinary catheters. Laminated sheets of instructions for reducing latex exposure and protocols for the management of anaphylactic reactions should also be available. Guidelines need to be tailored to meet local needs. The single most important precaution is the ready provision of latex-free gloves. Some manufacturers of surgical gloves have responded to the problem of latex allergy by producing 'hypoallergenic' gloves. These gloves are designed to overcome the problem of contact dermatitis due to chemicals used to vulcanise gloves and are not suitable for patients with latex allergy. Latex-free gloves are made of plastic. Unfortunately, the best of these are still inferior to latex gloves in terms of fit, flexibility and sensitivity, and this accounts for the continued preference for latex in surgical practice.

The management of the latex-allergic patient is important. Ideally, the patient should be nursed in a side room clear of latex and rubber products. It is important to ensure that all staff involved with the patient are fully aware of the patient's allergy and the information is posted on the patient's charts and identity band. Prior to surgery, prophylaxis should be given. Some anaesthetists advocate the preoperative administration of antihistamines and steroids for 24 hours and postoperative administration for 12 hours, and other anaesthetists are content to prescribe a single dose of antihistamine and steroids to be given with routine preoperative medication. The following regimen has few major disadvantages:

- Chlorpheniramine 10 mg i.v. 6-hourly
- Ranitidine 50 mg i.v. 8-hourly
- Hydrocortisone 100 mg i.v. 6-hourly
  The dosages should be adjusted for **children:**
- Chlorpheniramine
  Less than 1 year: 250 µg/kg
  1–5 years: 2.5–5.0 mg/kg
  6–12 years: 5–10 mg/kg
- Ranitidine 1.0 mg/kg
- Hydrocortisone 2.0 mg/kg
- Salbutamol nebulisers should be prescribed for patients with pre-existing asthma.

Patients who must undergo emergency or urgent surgery and who have had risk of latex allergy should receive the prophylactic medication as soon as is feasible.

The Association of Anaesthetists of Great Britain and Ireland produce guidelines for the **management of anaphylactic shock** and it is these instructions, which should be available in every operating theatre, that must form the basis of life-saving reactions.

Treatment includes the use of:

- Oxygen;
- Adrenaline (intravenous 0.5–1 ml increments 1:10 000); and
- Intravenous fluid support.

Anaphylactic reactions may become biphasic, with recurrence within 8–12 hours. For this reason, even if the patient's response to intervention is satisfactory, transfer to a critical care facility is warranted after a reaction. Mast cell degranulation can be confirmed with a serum tryptase level. This peaks 1–2 hours after the anaphylactic reaction. This is an important investigation for any patient who experiences otherwise unexplained perioperative cardiovascular collapse.

3

Trauma and Emergency Anaesthesia

Emergency orthopaedic anaesthesia is required in specific circumstances. Immediate resuscitation and surgery are often needed in patients with multiple trauma whilst urgent anaesthesia is required for the reduction of compound fractures and injuries in which fracture oedema, as in supracondylar fracture at the elbow, may result in nerve compression and arterial occlusion. Semi-elective surgery is carried out for fractures (e.g. neck of femur); experienced members of staff carry out surgery when the patient's condition is optimal during the normal working day.

Immediate Surgery – Major Trauma

Major trauma is the commonest cause of death in patients aged less than 40 years. Timely and appropriate resuscitation should prevent patients dying from the secondary consequences of their injuries – mainly head injuries and hypovolaemia. Following initial care, good subsequent management can reduce deaths from sepsis and organ failure.

Initial Evaluation

The prevention of hypovolaemic shock and neurogenic shock, after head and spinal cord injuries, combined with minimising the effects of the systemic inflammatory response syndrome and the prevention of infection, are the prime considerations following trauma. Systemic inflammatory response syndrome is diagnosed when any two of the following signs are present:

- Temperature >38°C or <36°C;
- Pulse >90/minute;
- Respiratory rate >20 breaths/minute or a $PaCO_2 > 4.3$ kPa; and
- WBC >12 000 cells/mm³ or < 4000 cells/mm³ or >10% immature band forms.

The management of the trauma patient is shown in Box 3.1. The initial aim is to look in a sequential order for immediately life-threatening injuries that kill.

Box 3.1   Management of the Trauma Patient

Primary survey and resuscitation
  Airway with cervical spine control
  Breathing – pneumothorax, cardiac tamponade, flail chest
  Circulation and haemorrhage control
  Disability – neurological function (AVPU or Glasgow Coma Scale)
  Exposure – prevent hypothermia
Secondary survey
  Continuous evaluation, cross match
  Further resuscitation and ?surgery
  Full examination – head to toe and front to back
  Medical history
  Investigations
  Plan for management
Definitive care

The patency of the airway can be assured by the use of routine simple devices such as the Guedel and, if a base of the skull fracture has been excluded, soft nasopharyngeal airways. In the unintubated patient, oxygen administered by a mask with an attached reservoir bag will provide an FIO_2 of as much as 0.85.

Assume that all patients with a blunt injury have a cervical spine injury. Immobilisation of the cervical spine by a semi-rigid cervical collar and sandbags and the use of a long spinal board virtually eliminate neck flexion. If intubation of these patients is required, it is performed using manual in-line stabilisation (MILS) of the neck but care is required, as excessive traction can distract a cervical fracture. There is debate as to whether intubation, should it be indicated, is performed with the patient awake or under anaesthesia. Coughing, bucking, raised intracranial pressure, bleeding, and laryngospasm can occur after a topical and a regional anaesthetic technique, and many anaesthetists prefer general anaesthesia using a rapid sequence induction technique with intubation aids, especially a gum elastic bougie, to assist tracheal intubation. Laryngoscopy can be difficult and should be performed by an experienced anaesthetist. Awake fibre optic intubation with adequate application of local anaesthetic agents to the mucosa above and below the vocal cords, performed by an experienced anaesthetist, is the ideal. However, few anaesthetists are sufficiently slick with this technique when rapid protection of the airway is required.

It is also important to assume a cervical fracture is unstable until appropriate radiological investigations (lateral, anterior–posterior and odontoid views) have been completed and reviewed by an expert.

Pneumothorax, whether it be open, tension or massive, requires chest drainage. A tension pneumothorax requires immediate decompression by the insertion of a large cannula placed through the second intercostal space in the mid-clavicular line. More permanently, a large chest drain should be placed in the fifth intercostal space in the mid-axillary line, with the drain connected to an underwater seal. A patient with a flail chest segment, which moves paradoxically with respiration, needs effective analgesia. This is best achieved by a thoracic epidural. The patient must also be watched carefully for underlying lung contusion.

As a rule, hypotension is caused by hypovolaemia, although the rarer causes pneumothorax, cardiac tamponade and, of course, hypoxia should never be forgotten. The source of haemorrhage must be established. Blood lose from fractures can be significant:

- Fractured femur – 3 units;
- Pelvic fracture (diagnosed by springing the pelvis on initial examination) – 3 units; and
- Tibial fracture – up to 2 units.

A pelvic fracture should be 'closed' by the immediate application of an external fixator. However, other occult causes of bleeding must not be overlooked – liver and splenic trauma can bleed heavily. It is a tragedy if abdominal injury is overlooked and, if in doubt, peritoneal lavage or laparotomy or ultrasound examination is indicated. Resuscitation involves warmed crystalloid or colloid replacement, initially at a volume 10–20 ml/kg, followed by blood. A central venous cannula is mandatory to give a guide to volume replacement. The patient should be kept warm by appropriate warming blankets.

Neurological examination is vital. The Glasgow Coma Scale (GCS) is used as an indication of central neurological damage. Box 3.2 shows the GCS in more detail. Localising signs and papillary reaction should be sought and noted. Sequential changes in the GCS score are a convenient way of assessing neurological progress. A GCS < 8 is serious, and often an indication for tracheal intubation.

The AVPU scale is a simple, rapid means for neurological assessment:

- A = alert,
- V = responds to vocal stimuli,
- P = responds to painful stimuli,
- U = unresponsive.

Box 3.2   The Glasgow Coma Scale

Response	Score
Best motor response	
Obeys commands	6
Withdraws from painful stimuli	5
Localises to painful stimuli	4
Flexes to painful stimuli	3
Extends to painful stimuli	2
No response	1
Best verbal response	
Orientated	5
Confused speech	4
Inappropriate words	3
Incomprehensible sounds	2
None	1
Eye opening response	
Spontaneously	4
To speech	3
To pain	2
None	1

The aim of the secondary survey is to obtain a full examination and history, and to plan safe investigations and further care. AMPLE is the useful mnemonic:

- A = allergies,
- M = medications,
- P = past medical history,
- L = last meal,
- E = event leading to injury and the environment.

Medical staff occasionally err in this area, and a patient requiring a laparotomy for intra-abdominal haemorrhage arriving at an isolated orthopaedic hospital is time delaying and life threatening. The patients requiring laparotomy need transfer to a general hospital environment for abdominal surgery first.

Initial trauma care also includes the careful titration of analgesia (intravenous morphine incrementally) in appropriate cases. This must not be forgotten.

Anaesthetic Techniques
The techniques of anaesthesia for major trauma cases are often compli-cated and it is mandatory that all monitoring lines are inserted rapidly

---

Box 3.3   Intubation Techniques

Remember manual in-line stabilisation in patients with suspected
  cervical spine fractures. Using the surgeon to provide cervical
  stabilisation frees up anaesthetic assistance and spreads responsibility.
Above the cords
  Blind intubation
  Nasal
  Using laryngeal mask
  Laryngeal visualisation
  Oral (± gum elastic bougie)
  Laryngeal mask with fibre-optic laryngoscopy
  Fibre-optic laryngoscopy
Below the cords
  Cricothyroid puncture
  Retrograde intubation
  Cricothyroidotomy
  Transtracheal ventilation
  Tracheostomy

---

and efficiently. Venous cannulae for fluid replacement and central
venous pressure measurement are necessary, as is direct arterial pressure
cannulation. Nasogastric tube insertion to allow gastric contents drainage
and urinary catheterisation to allow assessment of fluids and renal function is mandatory. In patients who have not been previously intubated, a
rapid sequence induction technique is necessary. Box 3.3 shows the intubation techniques available. Remember, intubation can be performed
under local or general anaesthesia.

Analgesia for major trauma is often provided by means of opiates
(intravenous morphine). Regional techniques are rarely used and epidural and spinal anaesthesia are inappropriate in 'unstable' or hypovolaemic states. Patients are often ventilated postoperatively until they
are warmed and stable.

Urgent Surgery

Some orthopaedic surgery needs to be done as soon as possible. The
classic examples are:

1. Compound fractures
   - Open fractures (the skin is broken) are highly susceptible to
     infection and therefore should be closed as soon as possible.
   - Osteomyelitis leads to huge problems, especially if a joint is
     involved in the fracture or if a plate is required to secure the fracture.

- Ongoing infection leads to unhealed fractures as well as ongoing general debilitation.
- These cases must be fixed under antibiotic cover as soon as possible, under either a suitable regional block or general anaesthesia using a rapid sequence induction technique.
2. Fractures with the risk of nerve compression and arterial occlusion. The classic example of this scenario is supracondylar fracture at the elbow in a child.
    - Firstly, children (and adults) do not empty their stomach after trauma and delaying surgery until the next morning does not guarantee that the child will have an empty stomach. Children are notorious for vomiting and aspirating stomach contents even 24 hours after their last meal.
    - Secondly, these fractures cause oedema at the fracture site and this can compress the arterial supply to the limb – no distal pulse is palpable. This results in distal limb ischaemia which, if not resolved, will lead to gangrene of the affected limb.
    - Surgery to reduce the fracture is necessary as soon as possible.
    - A rapid sequence induction technique is mandatory as part of the anaesthetic technique.

Semi-Elective Operations

Many patients undergo trauma from accidents, and most but not all can wait until the first available trauma list. An efficiently managed theatre suite will have a list available daily for this work. The list should be carried out by an experienced anaesthetist and surgeon. Simple fractures, dislocations and complex elderly cases can be managed this way. This allows for adequate fasting prior to anaesthesia and for the primary treatment of any concomitant medical conditions.

Debate about when the optimal time for surgery in the elderly trauma case exists. A patient with a fractured neck of femur requires being in optimal medical condition for surgery but unnecessary delays in this special group of patients can cause problems. Prolonged enforced bed rest results in debilitation, pain, chest infection and the development of bed sores in the elderly. Systemic analgesics provide only intermittent pain relief and cause confusion, vomiting and constipation. It is important not to delay surgery unnecessarily in this special group of patients.

The principles of anaesthesia are elucidated more completely in Chapter 4 but it is important to remember that surgery can be performed for all these operations under general or regional anaesthesia or a combination of both. Often, carefully balanced epidural anaesthesia is the method of choice, as good cardiovascular stability can be provided and the complications of general anaesthesia avoided.

Hip Fractures

Although most specialist orthopaedic hospitals do not have an Accident and Emergency department and, therefore, rarely see patients with a fractured neck of femur, it is the commonest injury on the trauma list in most district general hospitals. The main considerations for these patients are shown in Box 3.4.

Preoperative optimisation of these elderly patients has been shown to improve outcome, and surgery should be performed as soon as possible by an experienced team during the working day, with the patient in the best medical condition. Most fractures result from trauma but, as 80% of patients are aged over 75 years, many medical conditions can cause the patient to fall and a fracture result. Cardiac disease, e.g. Stokes Adams attacks, dysrhythmias, and neurological causes must be sought. Rarely renal disease, drugs, and electrolytic disorders also contribute to the condition.

Early appropriate fluid resuscitation and analgesia must be instituted but it must be remembered that opiates cause confusion, vomiting, and constipation. Immobilisation of the affected leg with lightweight skin traction provides considerable pain relief. Remember that many of these patients have poor nutritional status and, with immobility, are particularly at risk of developing pressure sores.

Hip fractures are of two types:

1. Intracapsular and subcapital fractures are associated with little preoperative blood loss. If the femoral head is undisplaced or minimally displaced, they can usually be fixed by percutaneous screws or pins. Significantly displaced subcapital fractures require hemi-arthroplasty

---

Box 3.4   Considerations for Patients with Hip Fractures

Optimal medical condition
Experienced team during normal hours
Elderly patients
Reason for the fracture – trauma or medical cause
Preoperative analgesia
Nature of surgery determines blood loss
Position on the operating table
Anaesthetic technique
Postoperative analgesia

or even total hip replacement (e.g. patients with rheumatoid arthritis or younger active patients);

2. Intertrochanteric fractures, where the preoperative blood loss is equivalent to that of a fractured femoral shaft (1–1.5 l) are usually fixed with a pin and plate device (e.g. dynamic hip screw or DHS). Aggressive but meticulous fluid replacement is required, taking into account the blood loss at the fracture site, oral intake and the fasting period.

Anaesthetic Management

With the exception of management by arthroplasty, hip fractures are reduced and fixed with the patient on an orthopaedic traction table (Hawley table). This limits the anaesthetist's ready access to the patient. Regional, general or a combination of both techniques is appropriate, and studies have shown little difference in terms of morbidity or mortality. General anaesthesia is associated with a shorter overall operative time but there is no significant difference between transfusion management, postoperative oxygen tension, postoperative confusion, or the incidence of myocardial infarction or stroke when general or regional techniques are compared. Given that there is little intrinsic benefit in employing a regional technique, there are a number of additional factors worth considering.

1. A fractured neck of femur is painful. Moving the patient into position for regional blockade makes the pain worse. Analgesia must be adequate and care must be taken to ensure that there are minimal respiratory complications from systemic opiates.
2. A minimally displaced subcapital fracture with a reasonable expectancy of the blood supply to the femoral head being intact may be completely displaced and the femoral head rendered avascular by positioning the patient for epidural or spinal injection.
3. Confusion and dementia are common in these patients. A confused patient who is awake may interfere with surgery and may resist arm restraint. Sedating the patient may lead to airway compromise.
4. Regional anaesthesia only provides a limited period of postoperative analgesia and then opiates will have to be used, which entails further side effects.

These facts are presented not to eschew a regional technique but to provoke planning the anaesthetic management to cope with all eventualities.

The surgical management of the patient with a fractured neck of femur is early mobilisation and prompt discharge. The anaesthetic management is integral to the success of this plan and the anaesthetist needs to be involved early, preferably as part of a multidisciplinary team caring for this large group of patients.

Repair of Brachial Plexus (and Other Peripheral Nerve Injuries)

Any neurological injury which results in a motor deficit is debilitating, but a complete supraclavicular lesion of the brachial plexus is a devastating injury. Its highest incidence is in young men – motorbike riders form a disproportionately large group. Iatrogenic injuries form another significant group, and neurological defect following vascular injuries or reduction of fractures and dislocations should not be assumed to be simple nerve contusion. If there was no pre-surgical intervention deficit, the surgeon should assume that the nerve has been divided and act accordingly. Anaesthetists too have been implicated and a small but steady group of patients present following nerve block attempts. The mean interval between nerve injury and referral to a specialist centre for peripheral nerve repair is over 6 months – such delays lead to a poor outcome.

The results of surgical repair are poor but improving. As well as the physical disability, patients also suffer from constant chronic pain. In patients with brachial plexus injuries, pain is more likely and more severe in injuries where the roots have been avulsed from the spinal cord, although traction injuries may produce a similar picture. The description of this type of pain is characteristic and at least 50% of patients report its onset from the moment of injury. The pain is described as crushing or burning and is chiefly in the forearm and hand over the anaesthetic area. Many of these patients attend chronic pain clinics and are opiate dependent. Surgery is warranted, as many of these patients state that the pain settles as muscle function recovers. Therefore, although early repair achieves a higher success rate, nerve grafting and transfer may be carried out months or years after the initial accident.

Anaesthetic Management

The anaesthetic management of these patients is important. Few brachial injuries occur in isolation, and patients frequently suffer other injuries:

- Fractured long bone >50%;
- Severe chest and head injuries – 15%; and
- 10% of supraclavicular and 25% of infraclavicular injuries also have a ruptured subclavian artery.

Other injuries, including those of the spine, must be sought and managed. Damage to the spinal cord from injury to the cervical and thoracic spinal column is not rare; potentially unstable skeletal injury is easily overlooked. The management of life-threatening injury must always take priority but early exploration, within hours of the injury, permits accurate diagnosis and simplifies the task of repair.

The aim of repair is to restore nerve function by nerve grafting or transfer. Surgery can be prolonged and may take 8–10 hours if avulsed nerves are reimplanted by grafting onto the spinal cord. Acute repair of injuries may involve vascular and spinal surgeons as well as orthopaedic surgeons. Vascular injuries may involve significant haemorrhage but on the whole even prolonged surgery involves minimal blood loss. The development of tissue compatible fibrin glues for joining nerves (rather than suturing) has shortened the operation considerably.

Specific considerations are as follows:

1. Neuromuscular blocking agents should be avoided, as the regular use of intraoperative nerve conduction studies is used to identify specific nerves and the sites of damage of the nerve supply to critical groups of muscles.
2. Surgery above or behind the clavicle may result in tears in the pleura which the surgeon may neglect to mention. Even in the absence of clinical signs, a postoperative chest X-ray may be warranted.

4

Joint Arthroplasty and Limb Surgery

Much elective and emergency orthopaedic surgery involves joint replacement and the endoscopic examination of joints, but there is a huge variety of operations, ranging from minor surgery such as toenail excision to massive revisional limb and joint salvage, involving all age groups.

Joint Replacement

Elective joint replacement is now an established treatment for end-stage disease of a joint for a variety of reasons:

- Osteoarthritis;
- Rheumatoid arthritis;
- Osteoporosis;
- Metastatic lesions; and
- Avascular necrosis.

Since the innovative work of Charnley in the 1960s on the development of total hip replacement, many advances in design and metallurgy have been developed. As a result of increased understanding of the biomechanical principles involved in the development of prostheses, and the use of acrylic cement to transmit forces between metal and bone, joint replacement has become increasingly successful. In the younger patient presenting for hip replacement with a history of previous trauma or congenital dislocation of the hip, custom-made prostheses are being increasingly used and are inserted without the use of cement. This, hopefully, will prolong the lifespan of the prosthesis.

Meticulous preoperative assessment must be performed. The majority of these patients are more likely to be older and have more serious medical problems. However, the elective nature of the surgery allows time for a thorough work-up, and effective treatment can be initiated if necessary. A history of the following conditions should be sought and, if current management is deemed inadequate, referral to the appropriate specialist undertaken:

- Hypertension;
- Myocardial infarction;
- Heart failure;
- Cerebrovascular disease; and
- Renal and liver insufficiency and pulmonary compromise.

Patients who have electrocardiograph evidence of ischaemia or a cardiac murmur require echocardiogram examination prior to surgery. Frequently, exercise tolerance is limited by joint pain before frank angina or overt breathlessness has been provoked: documentary evidence of adequate left ventricular function can be very reassuring when presented with an elderly patient on a vast range of medications!

A significant number of these patients will also be diabetic, and stringent control is essential in the perioperative phase. Diabetics are also at a greater risk of infection, and a prolonged course of antibiotic prophylaxis may be appropriate. Rheumatoid arthritis poses a major anaesthetic risk in joint replacement, and the major aspects of care are shown in Box 4.1.

Aortic stenosis is more prevalent in elderly patients and the presence of a systolic murmur in an elderly patient necessitates echocardiography to differentiate between sclerosis and stenosis. This is especially so in the presence of electrocardiographic evidence of left ventricular hypertrophy. The results will influence the choice of anaesthesia, perioperative monitoring and the need for postoperative HDU/ITU care.

Active infection is an absolute contraindication to joint replacement and any potential source must be eliminated, i.e. urine or dental infection. Aspirin and non-steroidal anti-inflammatory drugs are frequently the mainstays of analgesic treatment for arthritic patients and gastritis, anaemia and platelet dysfunction may occur. Accompanying medical and orthopaedic problems, together with side effects from drug treatment, make the rheumatoid patient considerably more difficult to treat. The salient problems associated with antibiotics, positioning, tourniquets, deep venous thrombosis prophylaxis, and cement are discussed in Chapters 1 and 2. The considerations and techniques available are summarised in Box 4.2.

Pre-medication is often desirable in this elderly and often nervous group of patients, and anti-hypertensive and other cardiac and respiratory medications should be administered as normal on the day of

---

Box 4.1   Problems with Patients with Rheumatoid Arthritis

Skeletal
  Instability of odontoid peg
  Atlanto-axial subluxation
  Restriction of mouth opening from temporo-mandibular joint arthritis
  Peripheral joint deformity causing difficulty in positioning of limbs
Respiratory
  Lung nodules
  Pleural effusions
  Pulmonary fibrosis
Nerves
  Exposure leading to inadvertent compression requiring padding
Drugs and their side effects
  Steroids
  Non-steroidal
  Immunosuppressants
  Gold
Skin fragility
  Adhesives can cause tearing and de-gloving
  Easy bruising
Other systems
  Normochromic normocytic anaemia
  Pericarditis
  Amyloid deposits affecting renal function

---

surgery. As an infected joint replacement is an absolute catastrophe for any patient, adequate antibiotic prophylaxis and attention to sterility is essential. Laminar flow air systems limit the quantity of airborne bacteria by controlling the flow of air in the operating theatre and should be routinely used for joint replacement surgery. Antibiotic prophylaxis should be administered well prior to skin incision to allow time for adequate tissue and bone penetration. *Staphylococcus aureus* and *Staphylococcus epidermidis* are the most commonly isolated pathogens and are sensitive to first-generation cephalosporins. Because isolated specialist orthopaedic hospitals do not have theatres that are used for bowel, urological or gynaecological surgery, infection rates for major arthroplasty are often less than those in general hospitals. However, there is no room for complacency as methicillin resistant *S. aureus* is increasing in all units.

Box 4.2   Considerations and Techniques for Joint Surgery

Intravenous access
Tourniquets
Duration of surgery – temperature homeostasis
Concomitant diseases
Drug therapy
Patient preference for type of analgesia and anaesthesia
Surgeon preference for type of anaesthesia
Emergency or elective in nature
Regional anaesthesia ± sedation
    Brachial plexus block for shoulder/elbow/wrist surgery
    Individual nerve blocks
    Intravenous regional anaesthesia
    Local anaesthetic infiltration
    Spinal/epidural/psoas block for hip/knee surgery
General anaesthesia
    ? Tracheal intubation
    Spontaneous or controlled ventilation
Patient position
Skin care and nerve damage
Infection
Methyl methacrylate cement
Deep vein thrombosis

Anaesthetic Techniques

Anaesthetic techniques for joint replacement are classified into regional or general anaesthesia or a combination of both. The advantages and disadvantages of each technique are shown in Boxes 4.3 and 4.4.

Sedation is often desirable in patients undergoing regional anaesthesia. The duration of surgery combined with operative noise as well as the lateral position for hip surgery makes patients restless and uncomfortable. Midazolam titrated in 1 mg aliquots is often used but can occasionally cause confusion and, in excess doses, can lead to loss of control of the airway.

Hip Replacement

This operation is normally carried out in the lateral decubitus position (or occasionally supine with a sandbag under the buttock) and attention to the position of intravenous cannulae and blood pressure cuffs is all-important. The blood pressure cuff should be placed on the upper arm to avoid inaccurate readings. There is no single ideal anaesthetic technique but general anaesthesia is still commonly used, the combined spinal epidural is becoming increasing popular and a general anaesthetic

---

Box 4.3   Advantages and Disadvantages of Regional Anaesthesia in Joint Surgery

Advantages
   No general anaesthetic risks
   Decreased blood loss
   Decreased risk of deep venous thrombosis
   Better immediate postoperative analgesia
   Regional block can be extended if indicated for prolonged
      postoperative analgesia
   Possible earlier mobilisation
   Decreased risk of respiratory infection
   Less vomiting
   Less mental confusion in the elderly
Disadvantages
   Surgeon preference
   Patient preference
   Complications of regional technique used, e.g. epidural
      hypotension, headache
   Contraindications to a regional technique
   Difficulty in performing blocks in the elderly

Box 4.4   Advantages and Disadvantages of General Anaesthesia in Joint Surgery

Advantages
   Faster induction
   Patient preference
   Surgeon preference
   Better cardiovascular control (often)
   Control of the airway
   Avoids the contraindications and complications of regional
      anaesthesia
Disadvantages
   Risks of general anaesthesia
   Slower recovery
   Slower mobilisation
   Increased vomiting
   Greater potential for postoperative confusion
   Increase risk of respiratory infection

---

in combination with an epidural is another option. Blood loss is less with regional anaesthesia than with normotensive general anaesthesia and there is better surgical field visualisation. The incidence of deep venous thrombosis is less with regional anaesthesia. With good surgical and anaesthetic technique, the requirements for blood transfusion should be lessened and, for most hip replacements, should not be necessary. Reaming of the femur and insertion of cement are often associated with sudden decreases in blood pressure, a decrease in the end tidal carbon dioxide concentration and a drop in oxygen saturation.

Epidural analgesia is excellent for managing postoperative pain but it is important to remember that there is an increased risk of requiring urinary catheterisation with this technique. Urinary catheterisation can lead to bacteraemia and there is an increased risk of joint infection. Gentamycin should be given on removal of the catheter to prevent infection as well. Patient-controlled analgesia is also used for postoperative analgesia but can cause vomiting, nausea, constipation and confusion in the elderly.

Knee Replacement

This operation is carried out with the patient supine and a tourniquet is usually used. Antibiotics should be administered at least 5 minutes prior to inflation of the tourniquet. Thorough attention to haemostasis by the surgeon following tourniquet release but prior to wound closure considerably lessens ooze postoperatively. When the tourniquet is released, acidic by-products of metabolism are released. These cause hypotension secondary to vasodilatation and negative effects on cardiac contractility. If the tourniquet is not released until the end of the surgery, the patient can experience pain from this cause alone on awakening.

Anaesthetic Technique

A regional technique that may be carried on into the postoperative period is an advantage as knee replacement is a very painful operation for the first 12 hours after surgery. The pain can be lessened by the use of a femoral nerve block when general anaesthesia is used alone. This will prevent the pain from quadriceps spasm.

Enlightened surgeons can be persuaded to infiltrate the back of the knee by injecting local anaesthetic through the posterior capsule into the two heads of gastrocnemius, which greatly enhances postoperative analgesia. The surgeon needs to be reminded to give the injection after the bony cuts have been made, prior to the cementing of the prosthesis, with the knee in extension. Injection is facilitated by providing a large spinal needle at the appropriate time.

Shoulder Replacement

Blood pressure monitors can be used on the nonoperative limb or the leg. If venous access is used on the same limb as the blood pressure cuff,

a non-return valve will prevent venous blood filling up the venous cannula when the pressure is being taken.

Anaesthetic Technique

Techniques vary for shoulder surgery. General anaesthetic techniques
vary from intubation with a reinforced tracheal tube and controlled
ventilation of the patient to spontaneous ventilation on an armoured
laryngeal mask in some self-selecting patients. Regional techniques are
commonly employed and, to ensure the shoulder is blocked, a supraclavicular approach is necessary. The most common is the interscalene
approach to the brachial plexus, which provides excellent intraoperative
analgesia, decreased blood loss and good muscle relaxation for any operation. As with all regional techniques which should be performed awake,
complications must be sought for and treated, the commonest being:

- Phrenic nerve palsy;
- Horner's syndrome; and
- Recurrent laryngeal nerve block.

Many shoulder surgeons have come to realise that adequate regional
analgesia extending into the postoperative period greatly improves the
chances of early postoperative mobilisation and physiotherapy for the
shoulder joint. This group of surgeons often insist on a regional technique being performed and are tolerant of the presence of indwelling
interscalene catheters during surgery.

Patient Position

Patient position is important for shoulder replacement. The patient is
positioned in a sitting position with a sandbag between the shoulders to
improve surgical access. The head must be secured, as traction often
pulls it off the head ring and dislodgement of the tracheal tube can occur
if it, likewise, is inadequately secured. The eyes should be well padded.
The surgical assistant may need constant encouragement to avoid resting his elbow on the patient's face.

Revision Arthroplasty Surgery

Revision surgery for joint replacement causes additional problems.
Perioperative hypothermia is a consideration, as the operations are
long by definition and appropriate patient warming devices should be
used. Blood loss is often considerable and occasionally a cell saver
can be used to help minimise blood transfusion. A cell saver is

contraindicated in patients with cancer or infection. In prolonged surgery, consideration should be given to care in a high dependency unit postoperatively.

Other Joint Procedures

Orthopaedic surgeons replace nearly all joints now and the above anaesthetic principles hold true for all joint surgery. Endoscopic work is also carried out on nearly all the joints small (wrist) and large (hip, shoulder, knee, elbow).

Arthroscopy

The indications for arthroscopy are both diagnostic and operative. Hip and ankle arthroscopies are primarily diagnostic procedures and are much less common than knee arthroscopy, which often involves an operative procedure, such as removal or repair of a torn meniscus, or reconstruction of torn ligaments. A torn labrum in a hip joint can be resected arthroscopically if the joint can be distracted on a fracture table. A small incision is made for the introduction of the arthroscope and the capsule of the joint is distended with sterile normal saline irrigating fluid to facilitate the view. For knee and ankle surgery, a tourniquet is usually used.

Anaesthetic Technique

Anaesthesia is usually carried out using general anaesthesia but any suitable regional technique can be used. In fit healthy patients, arthroscopic surgery is usually carried out as a day case. However, arthroscopic synovectomy is a painful procedure requiring admission for postoperative pain management.

Limb Operations

Osteotomy of both large and small joints is performed under both regional and general anaesthesia. All of these operations are painful in the postoperative phase for the patient. All carry the risk of infection and antibiotic cover must be given.

Muscle and tendon transfer operations are commonly performed on patients who have intercurrent arthropathies to facilitate better joint function. Position is important and care must be exhibited if the patient is being placed in the prone position, which can occur in tendo-Achilles surgery. Soft tissue operation is considerably less painful than bony resection and lends itself to local anaesthetic infiltration, unless the surgeon is concerned about peripheral nerve function.

5

Bone Tumours

The last 15 years have seen dramatic progress in the diagnosis and treatment of bone tumours. Advances in management mean that many malignant bone tumours are curable, but correct treatment requires an exact histological diagnosis, which can take up to 2 weeks from biopsy. Patients undergoing biopsy should be informed of this.

The classification of bone tumours is shown in Box 5.1.

Benign latent tumours grow slowly and stop, and have a tendency to heal spontaneously. Benign active lesions have a progressive growth pattern and a tendency to recur. Benign aggressive tumours are locally aggressive and have a tendency to recur unless widely excised. They do not metastasise. Malignant low-grade tumours are locally recurrent and have a small metastatic potential (<10%) whilst malignant high-grade tumours have rapid growth and a tendency to metastasise early.

Primary bone tumours (i.e. those originating from bone cells) are difficult to diagnose because of their rarity and may take up to 18 months to diagnose from the patient's initial presentation with a complaint to the general practitioner. In addition, some malignant bone tumours cannot be distinguished from their benign form by histology alone, and final diagnosis requires additional knowledge of the clinical history and X-ray appearance of the lesion. Thus, to ensure the accuracy and efficacy of bone tumour management, the surgeon, radiologist and pathologist have a joint responsibility in reaching a definitive diagnosis.

Primary bone tumours are less common than secondary (or metastatic) bone tumours and represent less than 1% of all tumours, but all are on the increase. If myeloma is included, more than 75% of all bone tumours are malignant. Because of the rarity of the condition, most bone tumours are managed by tertiary referral centres, which increases the expertise of the doctors responsible. For each patient, a management plan is devised involving biopsy, clinical staging and or definitive treatment plan which may involve the clinical oncologist and radiotherapist. Following definitive treatment, the patient will require regular scans to exclude local recurrence and lung metastases for many months (or years) afterwards.

Box 5.1   Classification of Bone Tumours

Primary bone tumours
  Benign
  Latent, e.g. non-ossifying fibroma
  Active, e.g. aneurysmal bone cyst
  Aggressive, e.g. giant cell tumour
  Malignant
  Low grade, e.g. parosteal osteosarcoma
  High grade, e.g. osteogenic sarcoma
Secondary bone tumours – breast, kidney, thyroid, lung, bowel, prostate
Soft tissue tumours
  Benign
  Latent, e.g. lipoma
  Active, e.g. angiolipoma
  Aggressive, e.g. aggressive fibromatosis
  Malignant
  Low grade, e.g. myxoid liposarcoma
  High grade, e.g. malignant fibrous histiocytoma

Patients with bone tumours may present at any age. The commonest diagnoses in relation to age are:

- Under 6 years – metastatic neuroblastoma and leukaemia;
- Between 6 and 15 years – Ewing's sarcoma; and
- Above 50 years – metastatic bone lesions.

All primary bone tumours are more common in males. Pain is often the presenting complaint due to expansion of or destruction of tissue in the bone, or pathological fracture, and night pain is pathognomonic. They may also present as an incidental finding on an X-ray done for other reasons, and occasionally are diagnosed late, having already metastasised to the lungs, the main site of metastatic spread of bone tumours. Occasionally, a bone biopsy is carried out under computerised tomography guidance under general anaesthesia. If a lung CT is necessary for staging, it can be carried out at the same time. However, this must be carried out before the induction of general anaesthesia as it can be impossible to distinguish between the patchy atelectasis caused by general anaesthesia and lung metastases.

Systemic symptoms constituting a grave prognosis include:

- Fever;
- Weight loss; and
- Anaemia, such as can occur with Ewing's sarcoma.

Box 5.2   Anaesthetic Considerations for Bone Tumour Patients

Late diagnosis
Metastases – haematogenous spread to lungs
Chemotherapy effects
Radiotherapy effects
Haemorrhage
Nature of surgery
Limb salvage cement reactions
Amputation – phantom limb pain
Hypothermia

Anaesthetic considerations relevant to the bone tumour patient are summarised in Box 5.2.

Oncology

Orthopaedic oncology involves the management of patients with primary tumours of bone, cartilage and related connective tissues and includes patients with metastatic disease from other primary sites. Chemotherapy and, to a lesser extent radiotherapy, or both are an integral part of the preoperative treatment in many of these patients and consideration of their many side effects is mandatory. Side effects are relevant to the anaesthetist, as different drug regimens are being used all the time. Some patients will be suffering acute systemic upset related to these agents when they arrive in the anaesthetic room. Some will have evidence of long-term toxicity. The side effect profile may vary but the principles are still the same and are shown in Box 5.3.

Haematological effects are the most common and myelosuppression occurs, resulting in leucopenia, anaemia and thrombocytopenia. A white cell count of less than $2.0 \times 10^{-9}/l$ is a contraindication to surgery because of the ongoing risk of infection, as is a platelet count of less than $100 \times 10^{-9}/l$, which can lead to excessive haemorrhage. Cancer may lead to a hypercoagulable state, and patients are at an increased risk of deep venous thrombosis. Any form of dysrhythmia may occur in relation to chemotherapeutic agents, and a baseline tachycardia is common.

More rarely, cardiomyopathy or pericarditis may occur, particularly in susceptible patients receiving high doses of doxorubicin. Doxorubicin, daunomycin and adriamycin can all cause acute cardiac toxicity resulting in congestive heart failure and arrythmias. They can also cause a dose-dependent decrease in left ventricular ejection fraction. Preoperative evaluation of these patients should include an electrocardiogram and an

---

Box 5.3   Side Effects of Oncology

Haematological
  Anaemia
  Leucopenia
  Thrombocytopenia
  Hypercoagulability
Cardiac
  Dysrhythmias
  Cardiomyopathy
  Pericarditis
Respiratory fibrosis
Nephrotoxicity
Hepatotoxicity
Neurotoxicity
Poor neutritional state
Poor venous access

---

assessment of cardiac ejection function in the form of an echocardiogram in at-risk patients.

Pneumonitis may occur following radiotherapy or chemotherapy with bleomycin. This pneumonitis leads to irreversible pulmonary fibrosis, which is aggravated by the administration of supplemental oxygen. It must also be remembered that bone tumours frequently metastasise to the lungs. The presence of a mediastinal mass or upper airway obstruction may be a contraindication to general anaesthesia.

Nephrotoxicity is a hazard following cis-platinum and methotrexate therapy, particularly in the underhydrated patient. Renal tubular damage may lead to problems with hyponatraemia, hypokalaemia and hypocalcaemia. This nephrotoxicity can be compounded by the use of non-steroidal anti-inflammatory drugs, and many oncologists would suggest that these drugs are avoided in patients receiving platinating drugs and methotrexate. It must be remembered that many bone tumour patients come to surgery between courses of chemotherapy, and even though renal function may still be normal at the time of surgery, subsequent nephrotoxic chemotherapy may precipitate irreversible renal failure in the presence of non-steroidal drugs.

Hepatotoxicity does occur and baseline preoperative liver function should be evaluated to include clotting studies.

Neurotoxicity also occurs. Vinca alkaloids and cisplatin can cause profound peripheral and autonomic neuropathies. If a regional technique or a local anaesthetic block is contemplated, the anaesthetist should be aware of the patient's preoperative neurological status, which must be documented in the notes prior to anaesthesia.

Venous access may be difficult or impossible in those patients who have had the chemotherapy administered through peripheral veins. Many patients will have a Hickman line in situ and maintenance of sterility in handling these lines in immunosuppressed patients is essential. It makes little practical sense to persist in attempting to site peripheral intravenous access to induce a distressed child who has a Hickman line and anaesthetists should familiarise themselves with the management of these lines and use them for induction.

These patients may often be malnourished due to the systemic effects of their primary tumour and the distressing emetic properties of chemotherapy. Patients often have angular stomatitis (which cracks and bleeds on laryngoscopy) and ulcerated oropharyngeal mucosa. Petroleum jelly applied to the mouth and the use of local anaesthetic spray to the oropharynx and larynx are a humane and noninvasive intervention. Alopecia is a side effect of chemotherapy that both male and female patients find particularly distressing and the provision of disposable theatre hats prior to leaving the ward is usually appreciated by all patients. Remember that significant heat loss occurs from the head and orthopaedic wool can be used to provide effective insulation perioperatively.

Surgical Procedures

Within the past two decades limb salvage procedures have proved safe and effective alternatives to amputation for many patients with bony and soft tissue sarcomas. This advance has been augmented by the use of prostheses that are specifically fabricated for musculoskeletal reconstruction. Soft tissue and muscle transfers are used to cover the resection site and to restore muscle power. Amputation of limbs unfortunately may still also be indicated. Disarticulations through both shoulders and hip joints are occasionally indicated and, for more aggressive or fungating tumours, palliative forequarter or hindquarter amputation may be necessary. The cosmetic effects of such mutilating surgery are often underestimated by the surgical team, and it frequently falls to the anaesthetist to deal with the patient's distress. Experienced anaesthetists should, therefore, do preoperative visits.

Soft tissue tumours of the pelvis, proximal femur and buttocks are sometimes treated by a hemipelvectomy. Each method of surgical management, amputation or reconstruction, has its own complications.

Surgical procedures may be long and arduous, with tissue planes obscured by radiotherapy.

Operative Anaesthetic Management

Haemorrhage during surgery of the bigger tumours can be torrential. Even experienced anaesthetists can underestimate the loss as it occurs. These cases require adequate wide-bore venous access and arterial and central venous pressure monitoring throughout. Rapid infusion systems must be available. Massive transfusion with all the attendant fluid shifts is common, as is the development of a coagulopathy. Platelets, cryoprecipitate, and fresh-frozen plasma need to be given early. As a result, ongoing bleeding is often a problem postoperatively, even in patients with normal clotting, and is due to large exposed raw areas of tissue following resection of tumour. Antifibrinolytic agents such as aprotinin or tranexamic acid may help reduce oozing in this phase. Although there are no trials on the use of activated factor VIIa in this type of surgery, there are individual case reports indicating that it may have a place in the reduction of blood loss in major orthopaedic surgery.

Customised massive prostheses may require large volumes of acrylic cement which may cause problems in these patients, especially in those in whom the blood volume is low. Severe hypotension, bradycardia, severe oxygen desaturation and cardiac arrest can occur.

Hypothermia is also an issue (and worse in those patients with chemotherapy-induced alopecia). Active warming is an integral part of anaesthetic management.

Anaesthetic techniques normally include both general and regional anaesthesia. The regional component can be used in the postoperative phase for analgesia. All these patients should be nursed in a high dependency or an intensive care unit setting postoperatively with ongoing haemodynamic and haematological assessment. Theoretically, the use of the thromboelastograph (TEG) both intraoperatively and postoperatively should help considerably in the active management of those patients who bleed. In practice, the system is slow in giving results and the entire picture will have changed long before you will have acted on the TEG result during surgery. It may have a more effective role in guiding postoperative transfusion strategy. Blood, fresh frozen plasma, platelets and cryoprecipitate may all need to be administered in large quantities in the postoperative period for up to 2 days. Peri- and postoperative blood salvage systems are contraindicated in patients undergoing tumour surgery for fear of haematogenous dissemination of malignant cells, although the manufacturers of these systems promote their use in bone tumour surgery. It is useful to develop the habit of contacting the transfusion laboratory the day before surgery to discuss the perioperative requirements. During surgery, the transfusion technician is the anaesthetist's best friend.

Management of Metastatic Disease Involving Bone

Primary breast, lung, prostate, renal, bowel, and thyroid tumours most commonly metastasise to bone, with the vertebral column being most commonly affected. The facts are that 60% of patients dying of breast cancer have metastatic involvement of the spine. Secondary bony deposits occur anywhere where marrow is present, especially in the axial skeleton and in the proximal humerus and femur. If the patient is well enough to withstand the surgery and anaesthesia, palliative fixation may be offered. Spinal stabilisation with instrumentation may prevent neurological deterioration or paresis. In the case of long bones, prophylactic fixation with nails or plates is an option and, where fractures have occurred, prosthetic replacement may be required.

Hypercalcaemia is a concentration of calcium greater than 2.5 mmol/l and is particularly associated with breast and lung tumours. More than 50% of patients who have elevated calcium levels on incidental findings have metastatic tumours in bone. The mechanism for producing hypercalcaemia is most commonly primary invasion of bone but may also be due to the stimulation of bone reabsorption by humoral substances which activateosteoclast activity directly (e.g. osteoclastic-activating factor) or indirectly (e.g. parathyroid hormone activating-related peptide). The clinical signs of hypercalcaemia are subtle and non-specific, and over 50% of patients with hypercalcaemia are asymptomatic. Symptoms are unrelated to the concentration of calcium in the blood. The symptoms are shown in Box 5.4.

Patients are often significantly fluid depleted and rehydration may require 4–6 l of crystalloid fluid. Steroids are useful in the

---

Box 5.4 Symptoms and Signs of Hypercalcaemia

Anorexia, nausea and vomiting
Abdominal pain
Polyuria, polydipsia
Depression, poor memory
Drowsiness, decreased consciousness level
Electrocardiographic signs – short QT interval, prolonged PR and
    T-wave changes

management of hypercalcaemia related to malignancy but require several days of administration before their benefit is apparent.

Secondary bone tumours present other problems because metastatic disease tends mainly to involve the older population. Surgery may be technically more difficult and take longer, and these patients, particularly those with spinal secondaries, have a tendency to bleed severely.

The frail elderly patients with disseminated malignant disease have a poor prognosis, both in their ability to tolerate prolonged reconstructive surgery (and anaesthesia) and in subsequent quality of life. Spinal surgery procedures in these patients are aimed at relieving pain and preserving neurological function. The decision to undertake surgical intervention is determined by the primary site of disease and the general condition of the patient, and consideration must be given to the patient's likely length of survival. The aim is to improve the quality of life. It is also important to fully involve the patient and the family in decision-making, as early postoperative mortality occurs not infrequently in this difficult group of patients.

6

Paediatric Orthopaedics

The word 'orthopaedic' derives from the Greek for 'straight child' and what is now called paediatric orthopaedics was the original reason for the development of orthopaedics as a separate surgical speciality.

Paediatric conditions form a minority of orthopaedic practice and more than 50% of paediatric anaesthesia is for trauma. Elective paediatrics presents the anaesthetist with a range of uncommon congenital and developmental conditions, which may include rare metabolic disturbances as well as anatomical and behavioural problems, as part of a complex syndrome or as isolated findings. The child who presents for a single surgical intervention may show a degree of interest and cooperation not seen in the child who has had multiple operations and knows he is due for several more! To compound the problem, the relatively small numbers of patients with a given condition means that there is a lack of consensus on how to treat them, and the same condition may be managed very differently by different departments.

Only the commonest paediatric orthopaedic conditions will be discussed here, but for any patient who has a rare syndrome underlying their presenting complaint, a literature search for associated problems, which may be of relevance to the anaesthetist, pays dividends! Experienced anaesthetists with good paediatric knowledge should undertake anaesthesia in this subspecialty.

Clubfoot (Talipes Equinovarus)
The incidence of congenital club foot is approximately 1:1000 live births and is twice as common in boys as in girls. The deformity is bilateral in 50% of patients and bilateral talipes is more likely to be associated with other congenital anomalies. Most cases are sporadic but families have been reported with the condition presenting as an autosomal dominant trait.

There are many theories regarding the underlying cause of talipes but the defect is probably secondary to soft tissue abnormalities at the neuromuscular level. Clinically, there is atrophy of calf muscles and the affected foot is smaller and narrower than the unaffected foot.

The three basic components of clubfoot are:

• Equinus;
• Varus; and
• Adduction deformities.

Each can vary in severity, and is usually accompanied by tibial torsion. The deformity is exacerbated by contractures of the soft tissues which resist passive realignment of the joint. If uncorrected, many other late adaptive changes occur in the bones with degeneration or spontaneous fusion of some joints. X-ray is an integral part of the evaluation of clubfoot.

Initial treatment includes passive stretching and splinting. Early tenotomy of the tendo-Achilles allows the heel to be brought down. Incision for tenotomy is a percutaneous procedure, but the tendon overlies the neurovascular bundle and therefore there is the potential for significant bleeding. Following induction of anaesthesia, the surgeon should infiltrate the site of the incision with local anaesthetic prior to surgery. If this done before the skin is cleaned and draped, it may have worked before the incision is made. There is considerable soft tissue stretching and manipulation of joints prior to cast application and the degree of patient discomfort is not reflected in the apparently insignificant surgical procedure. However, opiate analgesia is rarely required and satisfactory analgesia can be obtained with regular paracetamol and non-steroidal anti-inflammatory drugs (NSAIDs). The surgery often takes much less time than establishing anaesthesia for it.

Definitive surgery to achieve anatomical correction requires:

• Major soft tissue release;
• Tendon lengthening; and
• Osteotomies.

While tenotomies are carried out at 3–4 months of age, final surgery is usually performed so that subsequent serial casting is completed by the time the child is starting to stand (about an age of 1 year).

The problems of anaesthesia for club foot surgery are shown in Box 6.1. The procedure is performed with the patient prone, and tourniquet control is essential. Pressures of 150–200 mmHg are used.

Hyperthermia rather than hypothermia is often more of a problem as only a small part of the patient is exposed. This is painful surgery and caudal epidural blockade, either as a single shot or continuous infusion, provides safe and easy analgesia. Caudal catheters may be placed using a

---

Box 6.1   Problems of Anaesthesia for Club Foot Surgery

Age 3–18 months normally
Prone position
Airway secure
Intravenous cannula secure
Tourniquet
Temperature control
Postoperative analgesia

---

strict aseptic technique with the patient in the lateral or prone position. A 20-gauge intravenous cannula may be used as a guide for a 19-gauge epidural catheter. Faecal contamination of the catheter site and infection are theoretical concerns although, clinically, they do not appear to be a problem. A greater problem is displacement of the catheter because the child is more comfortable and therefore more active. Even when a continuous infusion cannot be used for postoperative analgesia, the catheter can be used for intermittent top-ups during long procedures. Initially, 0.5 ml/kg of plain bupivacaine 0.25% is injected, followed at 90-minute intervals with one-third to one-half of the initial dose. Perineural injection of lignocaine by the surgeon prior to wound closure prevents the sudden loss of analgesia when central neuraxial blockade wears off, and we have found this technique very useful. Adequate analgesia must be prescribed in anticipation of the block wearing off. Regular oral opiate and non-steroidal anti-inflammatory medication will be required for at least 48 hours, following which paracetamol and a NSAID should suffice. It is imperative that medication is given regularly and not as the need arises.

Developmental Dislocation of the Hip (DDH)

This was formerly called congenital dislocation of the hip and the term includes:

- Subluxation of the femoral head;
- Acetabular dysplasia; and
- Complete dislocation of the femoral head out of the acetabulum.

It is usually identified in the newborn during a routine examination. X-rays are unreliable under 6 months of age, and ultrasound screening provides an accurate and noninvasive diagnosis. Occasionally, MRI scanning is required to make the definitive diagnosis and general anaesthesia may be needed to keep the child still. In our unit we do not use sedation for this procedure. As the child reaches 6–18 months, the condition becomes more obvious, with a decreased ability to abduct the hip because of contraction of the adduction muscles.

The incidence of DDH is approximately 1:1000 live births, with the left hip and bilateral involvement being more common than the right hip alone. The disorder is more common in females and in breech delivery babies, with up to 1 in 35 female breech deliveries being affected. It is more common in firstborn children and a positive family history increases the risk to 10%. There is an association between DDH and talipes and other musculoskeletal anomalies. The aim of all surgery is to produce a congruent, stable hip joint.

The treatment of DDH is age-related and tailored to the specific pathological condition. In babies up to 6 months of age, the hip joint can normally be manually reduced and management is directed to stabilising the joint with the femoral head in the acetabulum, using a dynamic flexion abduction orthosis such as the Pavlic harness. This gives excellent results when appropriately applied, although a potential complication is avascular necrosis of the femoral head. In infants (6–18 months), reduction may be achieved after an adduction tenotomy without the need for formal open reduction of the hip joint but, if closed reduction fails, open reduction is indicated. Local anaesthetic infiltration by the surgeon provides adequate analgesia after adductor tenotomy. There is no bony division and the leg is subsequently immobilised by the application of a hip spica cast.

Caudal or lumbar epidural blockade provides excellent perioperative analgesia. Lumbar epidural catheters need to be removed before application of a hip spica cast. The application of a hip spica ensures immobility of the joint and considerably reduces analgesic requirements. Oral paracetamol and non-steroidal analgesics are suitable.

The delayed diagnosis of DDH is becoming less common because of the widespread screening of neonates. When it occurs, the child may require femoral and pelvic osteotomies and the surgical management is much more demanding. Femoral and pelvic osteotomies are required to produce a congruent hip joint in DDH, either individually or together. This is major surgery and can be associated with significant blood loss. Haemorrhage occurs as a result of the osteotomy and will continue until the osteotomy has been reduced and fixed. The necessity for blood transfusion is determined by the duration of this part of the operation.

Plaster of Paris Hip Spicas
The application of a hip spica cast is performed under general anaesthesia and is difficult and time consuming. The child is placed on a spica

frame: a board supporting the head and trunk of the patient with the pelvis supported by a narrow extension. The board is placed at the foot of the operating table with the child's legs projecting over the free edge. The hips are held flexed and abducted whilst plaster of Paris slabs are applied around the torso and legs, incorporating the board of the frame. There is little support for the head or trunk, and maintaining monitoring is difficult as leads frequently become detached. The completed cast extends from just below the nipple line to the ankle on the operated side and to the knee on the opposite side. During application of the plaster, a pad of cotton wool or gauze should be placed over the abdomen to allow for abdominal distension. Once the plaster has hardened sufficiently, the spica frame is manoeuvred out and the child repositioned on the operating table for the cast to be trimmed to accommodate nappy changes. Removal of the abdominal pad at this stage facilitates ventilation. The anaesthetist should ensure that the surgeon has confirmed that final X-rays show the femoral head to be in a satisfactory position before waking the patient.

Plaster of Paris is applied as wet slabs. The colder the water used, the longer the plaster takes to harden, but the time available to achieve satisfactory moulding is increased. In addition, the plaster heats up considerably during the setting process. A significant portion of the child's surface area is initially cooled then warmed and, when ambient temperature is reached, the child is still enclosed by a 'wet' plaster. As a result, there are wide fluctuations in temperature, and hypothermia may ensue unless the child is nursed in warm surroundings until the plaster is fully dried. Unless staff are complaining about the heat, the plaster theatre is not warm enough!

Epiphysiodesis

Limb length discrepancy is not simply a cosmetic problem; it is also a functional concern. Where there is a difference in leg length, the resulting gait is awkward for the patient, and the end result is often back pain. Differences in leg length may be idiopathic, or result from trauma, infection or asymmetrical paralytic conditions such as polio or cerebral palsy. Differences in leg lengths of fewer than 2 cm require no intervention. Ideally, lengthening of the short limb would be the optimum treatment but this is technically difficult and prone to complications.

Epiphysiodesis is a percutaneous technique which involves obliteration of the epiphyseal plate through small incisions. Careful timing and consideration of the final height of the knee are important. Epiphysiodesis of both the distal femur and proximal tibia may be required. This is a relatively minor procedure with no blood loss and little postoperative analgesia is required.

Slipped Upper Femoral Epiphysis

This condition predominantly affects obese boys between the ages of 12 and 15 years. The incidence is approximately 1:10 000 and the lesion is bilateral in 30% of cases. It is not a feature of any particular syndrome but has been reported in association with Down's syndrome and hypothyroidism. The condition is of importance to the anaesthetist because lumbar epidural or spinal anaesthesia are relatively contraindicated because, when the patient is positioned prior to the insertion of the regional technique needle, complete displacement of the epiphysis can occur and destroy the blood supply of the epiphysis. If there is any contraindication to general anaesthesia, the situation must first be discussed with the surgeon.

Cerebral Palsy

The term cerebral palsy is used to cover a range of neuromusculoskeletal abnormalities thought to be due to hypoxia in the perinatal period. It has an incidence of 6:1000 live births. The child may be of normal intelligence, have significant mental impairment or have global developmental delay. Muscle spasticity is due to central neurological dysfunction. Muscle spasm results in contractures, and surgical intervention is aimed at releasing, lengthening or transferring tendons, and releasing or fusing joints to achieve a pain-free useful limb. Some children require repeated hospital admissions for multiple bilateral procedures. These children vary in their ability to cooperate and, even with children of normal intelligence, communication with strangers may be difficult. The presence of a parent or main carer may be invaluable in keeping the child calm in both the anaesthetic and recovery rooms.

Induction and anaesthesia are tailored to the individual child and procedure, but it is worth remembering that there is no contraindication to the use of suxamethonium, as significant potassium flux does not occur and there is no greater incidence of malignant hyperthermia than in the population at large because the lesion is of central neurological origin.

Postoperative analgesic requirements may be difficult to determine in children with communication problems. A continuous caudal or lumbar epidural infusion can be helpful for lower limb procedures as spasticity is reduced. Nevertheless, the postoperative period can prove a challenging time for both patient and carer.

Congenital Torticollis

This condition, also called 'wry neck', is of unknown aetiology. Up to 20% of cases are associated with DDH (see above). It is due to fibrosis within the sternomastoid muscle and produces a twisting of the neck and an unnatural position of the head. A mass is often palpated in the belly of the muscle (more commonly on the right side than the left) either at birth or within the first 2 weeks. The mass attains maximal size within the first 2 months and diminishes within 1 year. If there is a failure of the mass to regress, permanent fibrotic changes occur within the muscle. Because of the tendency to resolve, the initial management is conservative and involves gentle manipulation and careful adjustment of the sleeping position. Optimum age for surgical correction of the deformity is 1–4 years. Failure to treat the condition can result in permanent asymmetry of the face and skull and, if severe, of the ipsilateral shoulder.

Surgery involves tenotomy through an incision parallel to the medial end of the clavicle. Local anaesthetic infiltration by the surgeon provides excellent analgesia into the postoperative period and complications are rare.

Juvenile Chronic Arthritis

There are many causes of childhood arthritis, which are shown in Box 6.2.

Children with chronic juvenile arthritis form an important group of patients and present to anaesthetists in the district general hospital environment. Surgery is aimed at maintaining joint mobility, and it is important to remember that 40% of these children have more than five joints involved and up to 10% have systemic involvement (Still's disease). It is also important to remember that the cervical spine is often involved. Many patients present at a relatively young age for cervical stabilisation

---

Box 6.2   Causes of Childhood Arthritis

Trauma – sports injury, non-accidental injury
Viral infection – rubella, mumps, chicken pox, parvovirus
Bacterial (infective) – *Haemophilus, Staphylococcus, Mycobacterium tuberculosis*
Bacterial (reactive) – beta haemolytic streptococcus, enteropathic
Idiopathic – juvenile chronic arthritis
Autoimmune rheumatic disease – Henoch-Schonlein purpura, dermatomyositis, SLE
Malignancy – leukaemia, lymphoma
Haemophilia – haemarthroses

and fusion. This, in addition to temporo-mandibular joint involvement, can make intubation difficult. Many children also have symptoms of acid reflux as a result of steroidal and non-steroidal anti-inflammatory medication. Premedication should start 24 hours prior to surgery with a proton pump inhibitor such as lansoprazole or omeprazole.

The patients often have a daily spiking temperature, and can have lymphadenopathy, hepatosplenomegaly, and polyserositis, e.g. pericarditis. Patients who are known to have daily spiking temperatures should not have surgery postponed, but elective surgery is best performed when the disease is quiescent. Some children will have latex allergy. It must be remembered that mononeuropathies occur as a result of the disease and patients must be positioned carefully.

Septic Arthritis

This is a condition of infancy with the highest incidence between 1 and 2 years. It is a surgical emergency because destruction of the growth cartilage occurs rapidly and irreversibly. Other infection, such as otitis media, upper respiratory tract infection or infected skin lesions, such as paronychia, may precede septic arthritis and are thought to be the infective source, although no source may be identified. The hip is most commonly affected and *Staphylococcus aureus* and *Haemophilus influenzae* are the commonest infecting organisms. The child has usually been unwell for 1 or 2 days and presents with a high fever and evidence of systemic toxicity. Gastric emptying will have been slowed and the patient is often dehydrated as a result of reduced oral intake and pyrexia. Atropine is relatively contraindicated because of the risk of increasing the pyrexia further, and fluid resuscitation peri- and postoperatively is vital. Increased gas flows may be required during anaesthesia as the hypermetabolic state increases carbon dioxide production. Parenteral antibiotics will be required for a few days, and a second definitive intravenous cannula may be more easily established after fluid resuscitation whilst still under anaesthesia. The drainage procedure itself affords considerable pain relief as will the immobility achieved by splinting. The associated bacteraemia is a relative contraindication to epidural anaesthesia.

Obstetric Brachial Plexus Injuries

The incidence in the UK of obstetric brachial plexus injuries (OBPI) is not known, as there is no central registry, but published figures from other countries suggest a range of 0.1–4.0% of live births.

Two groups of children were identified as being particularly as risk: the heavy baby and the breech baby. The direct cause of the lesion is the forced separation of the forequarter from the axial skeleton by obstruction at the narrowest point of the birth canal. When the shoulder is forced downward the spinal nerves are stretched and the 5th and 6th cervical nerves are prone to rupture. This injury probably occurs as a result of shoulder dystocia, and babies with a birth weight of over 4.5 kg are at risk, with increased birth weight correlating with the severity of the injury; this is unsurprising, as the proportion of babies presenting with shoulder dystocia also increases with birth weight. When there is obstruction to breech delivery, it is in an upward direction with injuries occurring to the 7th cervical and 1st thoracic nerves. Involvement of the phrenic nerve is a dangerous complication and may call for urgent plication of the diaphragm.

The lesions may be partial or complete, transient or permanent and are classified as shown in Box 6.3.

As a result of the neurological deficit, there is usually limb length disparity ranging from 2% in Group 1 to 20% in Group 4. The management of OBPI depends on the degree of injury. Most children progress to at least useful neurological recovery, and initial management is watchful optimism. The aim of surgery is to encourage nerve growth through

---

Box 6.3   Classification of Obstetric Brachial Plexus Injuries

Group 1
C5 and C6 damage causes paralysis of deltoid and biceps. Full
  spontaneous recovery occurs within 2 months in 90% of cases.
Group 2
C5, C6 and C7 damage causes paralysis of extension at the elbow,
  wrist and fingers but long flexors of the fingers work. Full
  spontaneous recovery occurs in 65% between 3 and 6 months.
  Serious defects persist in the other 35% of children.
Group 3
Paralysis is more or less complete with only some flexion in the
  fingers being apparent at birth. Fewer than 50% recover
  spontaneously. There is impaired function at the shoulder and
  elbow and deficient forearm rotation. Twenty-five per cent fail
  to recover wrist and finger extension.
Group 4
The whole plexus is involved, with paralysis being complete. No child
  makes a full recovery. Horner's syndrome is apparent and the
  spinal nerves have been avulsed from the spinal cord. The cord is
  damaged in 2% of cases, and presents as delayed and unsteady
  walking.

nerve grafting. Infants with a complete lesion may undergo surgery after 1 month; incomplete lesions undergo surgery at around 3 months.

Anaesthesia for this surgery is therefore undertaken only by those who are experienced in anaesthetising this age group. By definition, many of these babies are fat and intravenous access takes time and skill. Nerve grafts are harvested from the injured upper limb using the medial cutaneous nerve of the forearm, superficial radial nerve and cutaneous division of the musculo-cutaneous nerve. Occasionally, the sural nerve is harvested and this involvement of the lower limb further impedes intravenous access. The clavicle may be divided during exploration of the brachial plexus and the pleura may be torn. Following nerve grafting, the infant is immobilised for 4 weeks in plaster of Paris splint, controlling movement of the head and neck and damaged upper limb. The postoperative presence of splinting restricts movements of the cervical spine and access to the jaw. Most anaesthetists favour extubation when the child is awake. Attempts to reintubate can be difficult, but a laryngeal mask can secure the airway in a crisis. The splint must be carefully applied so that the mother can continue to feet the child without undue difficulty and to clean the skin around the neck and chest.

The commonest and most significant secondary deformity in OBPI are:

• Medial rotation contracture; and
• posterior dislocation of the shoulder.

Later surgery may be required to improve function in 30% of OBPI with residual neurological deficit, particularly when there is involvement of C5 and C6 nerve roots. The best treatment of this secondary defect is prevention by regular and frequent physiotherapy. Surgical intervention involves muscle transfers about the shoulder, and the deformity occurs as a result of muscular imbalance in the growing limb. The deformity therefore varies from child to child and is not necessarily related to age. However, the deformity is progressive and there is a spectrum from medial rotation contracture to complex dislocation of the shoulder. Children in this group present at any age from 1 year to puberty. The majority of cases require soft tissue procedures only, and infiltration with local anaesthetic solution by the surgeon and perioperative opiate analgesia often suffice into the postoperative phase.

Regional neurological blockade is inappropriate in this patient group, not least because perioperative nerve conduction studies may need to be carried out. Residual neuromuscular blockade may also interfere with nerve conduction studies and may need to be reversed during surgery.

Occasionally, osteotomy of the glenoid is required. Postoperatively, the affected limb is immobilised for 6 weeks in a spica surrounding the thorax, with the arm held in lateral rotation. Plaster of Paris splinting for this procedure does not interfere with the anaesthetist's access to the airway.

7

Acute and Chronic Spinal Injury

Acute Injury

The precise epidemiology of acute spinal injuries is difficult to ascertain, since accurate statistics are not available. Spinal injury is not a notifiable condition and, in the majority of patients, it will be one of multiple injuries. The incidence of spinal injuries in the United Kingdom is estimated to be in the region of 20 per million of the population per year.

Traumatic causes of spinal injuries include:

- Road traffic accidents;
- Falls and sporting injuries; and
- Gunshot wounds and assault.

Road traffic accidents, with motorcycle accidents predominating, are the commonest cause, therefore the spinal injury population is predominantly male and young. A significant number of children suffer spinal injuries, especially as pedestrians involved in vehicle accidents. Falls and sporting injuries, particularly recreational diving and horse riding, form a major contribution to the traumatic causes of spinal injuries, and there is an increasing incidence of cases occurring as a result of gunshot wounds and assault.

Nontraumatic causes include:

- Vascular pathology, such as occurring secondary to aortic aneurysm surgery;
- Infection (with tuberculosis reappearing);
- Tumour, mainly metastatic from breast, haematological, prostate cancer; and
- Disc prolapse.

At the beginning of the 20th century, mortality associated with acute spinal injury was thought to be in excess of 80%. With improvements in acute and long-term care, there has been a dramatic decline in this figure. Many trauma patients will die at the scene of the injury due to multiple traumas but, for those spinal-injured patients that are hospitalised, the mortality figures quoted are between 2% and 20%. This reduction in mortality has led to an increasing population of chronic spinal cord injured patients, which in the United Kingdom is estimated, at present, to be 35 000–40 000 people. Box 7.1 shows the considerations related to these patients.

The spinal column can be thought of as having three columns: the posterior, middle and anterior columns. Flexion injury will maximally disrupt the posterior column and extension injury will maximally disrupt the anterior column. Disruption of two or more of the three columns will result in overall instability of the spine.

Spinal column injuries may be stable or unstable. Unstable injuries without cord damage can easily progress to spinal cord injury, and cord injury already present can be further extended if these cases are inexpertly managed. Stable injuries may be managed either conservatively by prolonged bed rest or by surgical fixation. Some spinal units favour surgical fixation over conservative management, citing the advantages of early mobilisation, and prevention of the development of future spinal deformity in the form of kyphosis or scoliosis. It may also reduce the incidence of syrinx formation that can lead to late neurological deterioration.

Spinal cord injuries can be complete, with total loss of neurological function below the lesion, or incomplete, with preservation of some neurological function. The final neurological deficit may not be clear until up to 1 year after injury. The cervical spine is the most common site of spinal column injuries, because it is the most mobile and the least

---

Box 7.1   Considerations in Acute Spinal Cord Injuries

Aetiology
Stability of the spine
Degree of loss of neurological function
Early management
Timing of surgery
Cardiovascular instability
Pulmonary oedema
Respiratory inadequacy
Gastrointestinal
Urinary
Spasticity
Skin
Temperature
Intubation problems
Maintain best cord perfusion conditions – blood pressure, no
   hypoxia, normocarbia

supported part of the spine, resulting in a natural vulnerability. Other common sites of damage are the thoraco-lumbar and the cervico-thoracic junctions, as a result of the junction between the rigid thoracic spine and the flexible lumbar or cervical spine.

Vascular Supply to the Spinal Cord

The spinal cord has a rather tenuous blood supply from three arteries, each supplying a specific territory of the cord. The anterior spinal artery arises from the vertebral arteries, with important contributions from the radicular vessels and supplies the anterior two-thirds of the cord. The two posterior spinal arteries arise from the posterior inferior cerebellar arteries and supply the posterior third of the cord.

Cord perfusion pressure is equal to the mean arterial blood pressure minus the cerebrospinal fluid pressure. It is subject to a degree of autoregulation but this is not preserved in the face of spinal cord injury. There is some alteration in blood flow relating to the partial pressure of carbon dioxide in arterial blood, with hypercapnia resulting in vasodilatation of the spinal vessels and hypocapnia causing vasoconstriction. Normocapnia or mild hypocapnia probably provides the best balance between vasodilatation and vasoconstriction, thus optimising cord perfusion and minimising oedema formation. The spinal cord is metabolically very active; therefore, a fall in perfusion pressure or hypoxaemia will rapidly produce ischaemic damage, triggering a biochemical cascade of reactions, with membrane disruption and cell death which will further compromise cord function.

Cord Injury

Damage to the spinal cord can be discreet, as from a piece of bone, or diffuse, as from a large haematoma, and may be described as primary and secondary.

Primary Injury

The initial damage is described as the primary injury. It is associated with vessel damage, local haemorrhage, vasospasm and ischaemia at a cellular level. This leads to multiple pathological processes culminating in secondary injury. Neural dysfunction occurs as a result of the traumatic disruption that takes place during primary injury and also as a result of the cell damage and death attributable to the secondary injury.

Secondary Injury

The secondary injury is caused by the generation of biochemical cascades associated with the acute inflammatory response, producing oedema, neuronal damage and death above and below the level of the primary injury. Neuronal function is preserved provided that perfusion is maintained through these areas until the oedema resolves.

Cardiovascular Changes Associated with Acute Spinal Cord Injury

The sympathetic chain runs from T1 to L2 with some variation, and sympathetic innervation is the principle influence on vasomotor tone. At the moment of injury to the spinal cord, there is thought to be a massive discharge of the sympathetic chain leading to vasoconstriction with consequent hypertension and dysrhythmias. If sympathetic stimulation is prolonged, there is a possibility of myocardial ischaemia and failure. There may also be disruption of pulmonary capillary endothelium, and pulmonary oedema may follow.

After spinal cord injury, patients may present with spinal shock syndrome. This is characterized by a period of flaccid areflexia in the muscles below the injury level. The consequent decreased systemic vascular resistance and increased venous capacitance leads to venous pooling and hypotension. If the cord is damaged at a low level, there will be enough functioning sympathetic innervation above the injury to compensate and blood pressure will be maintained. Injury at around T4 to T6 or higher leads to bradycardia, and decreased myocardial contractility may occur due to loss of the sympathetic innervation of the heart.

Parasympathetic supply via the vagus continues unopposed and patients with high injuries will be persistently bradycardic. Repeated doses of atropine or glycopyrrolate or temporary pacing may be required. An interesting point to note, however, is that even in high cervical spine injury, patients may still generate a tachycardia in response to hypoxia and hypercapnia. This response is most probably mediated by vagal inhibition rather than by sympathetic activation.

These vasodilated, hypotensive, bradycardic spinal cord injured patients should be assessed carefully for hypovolaemia. If there is no evidence of hypovolaemia and their haemodynamic status is secondary to vasodilatation, fluid will not improve their hypotension. They may already be at risk of developing pulmonary oedema as a result of the alveolar disruption that occurs with the severe pulmonary hypertension at the time of injury.

Central venous pressure monitoring may be unhelpful in these cases due to the virtual absence of peripheral resistance and dilated venous capacitance giving low values even in the face of fluid overload.

Oesophageal Doppler or pulmonary artery catheter monitoring may be more useful. The ultimate aim of management is to:

* Maintain perfusion;
* Avoid hypoxia; and
* Minimise the extent of secondary injury in the spinal cord.

Patients will be liable to postural hypotension in the first few weeks after injury. Gradual adaptation takes place over the long term.

Respiratory Physiology of Acute Spinal Cord Injury

The muscles involved in breathing are primarily the diaphragm and intercostals muscles, with small but important contributions from the accessory muscles; sternomastoid, platysma (both supplied by cranial nerves and therefore not affected by a spinal injury), and the scalenes (supplied by C4 to C8). The abdominal muscles (innervated by T10 to L2) have a significant role as expiratory muscles. Mid or high thoracic injuries produce both an inability to cough and intercostal muscle paralysis that leads to an increase in chest wall compliance, decreased vital capacity and decreased functional residual capacity. Untreated, this will progress to basal atelectasis and decreased pulmonary compliance. The resultant increased work of breathing and impaired gas exchange may cause respiratory failure, especially if there are additional rib fractures or lung contusions associated with the spinal injury.

Low cervical injuries abolish cough and all chest wall tone. Satisfactory respiratory function may be maintained using diaphragm alone, but respiratory failure often develops rapidly.

Injuries at C4 or C5 may leave enough diaphragmatic and accessory muscle function to maintain ventilation temporarily until ascending cord oedema removes diaphragmatic function. Injuries at C1 or C2 require immediate initiation of assisted ventilation to maintain life.

It follows, therefore, that monitoring respiratory function is essential with cervical or high thoracic injury as patients may develop respiratory failure several days later. In practice, this means that the patient who shows no evidence of respiratory compromise in the first few days after injury may well need ventilation later or following surgery and may be ventilator dependent for several days or weeks. If no intensive care bed is available, do not proceed with surgery in the hope that as, the patient was coping before, he or she will cope afterwards. The simplest and universally available measure of respiratory function is the vital capacity. In general, if an adult patient has a vital capacity of under 1l, the probability of respiratory failure is high, and a vital capacity that is approaching the patient's predicted tidal volume is an indication for ventilatory support. Serial arterial blood gases will be helpful in monitoring carbon dioxide retention. Monitoring respiratory rate and pulse oximetry in these patients may not reveal impending respiratory failure.

The management of respiratory failure due to cord injury depends on the level of injury, pre-existing lung pathology and many other factors. Basic management includes humidified oxygen, standard respiratory physiotherapy techniques and constant monitoring. Respiratory failure may be managed with continuous or intermittent noninvasive ventilation until the patient has recovered from the initial insult. Patients with significant respiratory impairment or persistent sputum retention are likely to require tracheal intubation.

Patients with respiratory failure after spinal cord injury who require a tracheostomy need a surgically fashioned tracheostomy. There is no place for siting percutaneous tracheostomies in this group of patients, even when the tracheostomy is likely to be temporary. Remember that these patients may require several temporary tracheostomies over the course of their lifetime.

Spasticity

Immediately after a spinal cord injury, the clinical picture is of a lower motor neurone lesion with flaccidity and areflexia. This may convert to spasticity and hyper-reflexia between 6 days and 6 weeks after the injury. The increased muscle tone may be associated with muscle spasms that are sometimes very severe and require treatment with agents such as baclofen and dantrolene. Active physiotherapy should be performed to reduce the risk of developing contractures.

Gastrointestinal Tract

Stress ulceration may occur during the acute phase of the injury. Ileus, as a result of sympathetic disruption, and occasionally retroperitoneal haematoma, is common, and may be severe. Enteral feeding as early as possible, sometimes with gastrostomy or jejenostomy formation, is advisable, remembering that the symptoms of peritonitis may be masked by the absence of normal sensation. Gut mobility may not respond to prokinetic drugs, and the lower bowel activity is lost, so aperients may be needed. Disorders of swallowing with silent aspiration are being increasingly recognised in high cervical cord injuries, particularly associated with anterior cervical spine surgery.

Urinary Tract

Spinal-injured patients require initial catheterisation with a silicon catheter until further urinary management is contemplated. Urinary tract infections should be treated early and aggressively.

Temperature

Patients may become effectively poikilothermic since they cannot alter muscle tone, shiver, vasoconstrict, vasodilate or sweat. Therefore, their temperature should be monitored closely and actively controlled.

Skin

Lack of sensation, lack of movement, absence of cutaneous circulatory control, poor nutrition with a low albumin and poor healing ability all contribute to a high likelihood of development of pressure sores. These patients should thus be nursed with meticulous pressure area care as the development of sores can significantly delay mobilisation, rehabilitation and discharge.

Early Management of the Acute Spinal Injured Patient

On presentation to hospital, patients with an acute spinal injury should be treated as any trauma patient according to the principles outlined in Chapter 3. Intubation should also be performed using these principles. Suxamethonium can be used immediately. Following spinal cord injury and acute muscle denervation, acetylcholine receptors increase in number and spread from the end plate to the surface of the affected myocyte. This occurs over a few days and lasts an indeterminate time. Suxamethonium should be avoided 48 hours after injury. When suxamethonium is administered, there is depolarization throughout the entire muscle surface membrane instead of just at the end place, causing a large ionic flux and a possible fatal release of potassium ions. The amount of muscle mass involved should be taken into consideration. Basically, the higher level of the cord injury, the shorter the window in which suxamethonium can be safely used. The time at which it is considered safe to use suxamethonium is variously quoted as 6 weeks to 6 months following injury. Considered logically, if muscle tone and spasticity have developed, then muscle innervation has returned and the end plate receptor population may have decreased, enabling the safe use of suxamethonium.

The unconscious patient should be treated as having a spinal injury until proved otherwise. Ten per cent of spinal injuries occur at more than one level and many are difficult to identify on X-ray. This is especially true for injuries to the upper thoracic spine but, in these cases, there may be associated rib, sternal or clavicular fractures. The force required to disrupt the thoracic spine is considerable. Thoracic spine injuries may be associated with injury to the heart and great vessels. A wide mediastinal shadow on chest X-ray may warrant aortic arch angiography to exclude dissection, and the angiography should be carried out in a centre that can manage the dissection.

A spinal cord injury with deteriorating neurological function must be treated as a surgical emergency and decompressed urgently to minimise the extent of the damage to the cord. The results in terms of neurological recovery can be significant. Spinal surgery should be performed when the patient is haemodynamically stable, but as soon as possible after the injury. Beyond 3 weeks post-injury, the healing process may make surgery technically difficult. Transferring these patients from bed, to trolley, to operating theatre table requires expertise and manpower. There is no place for making do. Even if the injury has caused a complete lesion, if it is unstable you can make it worse.

The Role of Steroids in Acute Spinal Injury

There have been three National American Spinal Cord Injury Study (NASCIS) projects which have attempted to find a pharmacological solution to reducing the neurological damage caused by spinal cord injury. Methylprednisolone seems to be beneficial when compared to placebo, naloxone and tirilizad (a steroid like drug), and it appears to act by reducing the effects of the inflammatory reaction around the area of the damaged cord. The degree of improvement is minimal and there has been criticism of the statistical analyses employed. Nevertheless, currently in the USA, the failure to administer steroids is grounds for litigation.

Methylprednisolone should be used according to the guidelines in Box 7.2 and it should be started within 4 hours of injury. If commenced

---

Box 7.2   Guidelines for Steroid Use in Acute Spinal Injury

Ideally give within 4 hours of injury for 24 hours
Methylprednisolone intravenously as a bolus followed by an
   infusion
Bolus dose 30 mg/kg over 15 minutes
Infusion at 5.4 mg/kg/hour 45 minutes after the bolus dose
Guide to administration: Methylprednisolone is presented in
   1 and 2 g vials as a dry powder with water for injections as a
   diluent which can be further diluted in normal saline.

between 4 and 8 hours after injury, it should be given for 48 hours. If the patient presents after 8 hours, steroids should not be given.

Methylprednisolone has the side effects of all corticosteroids and it is important to remember that diabetes mellitus may be precipitated or exacerbated. Respiratory tract infections are also more common. Acne may also be caused and mental disturbances in the form of euphoria, hallucinations or psychosis can occur.

Anaesthesia for Chronic Spinal Injuries

There are an estimated 35 000–40 000 patients with chronic spinal cord injuries in the United Kingdom. They present for any type of surgery but in particular genito-urinary, orthopaedic and neurosurgical procedures.

Spinal cord injury is categorised into three phases:

1. The first phase is from the immediate injury. If the injury involved the sympathetic outflow, there is a sudden discharge which results in vasoconstriction, hypertension and dysrhythmias.
2. The second phase of 'spinal shock' lasts from a few days and up to 8 weeks. There is areflexic flaccidity distal to the cord injury. Hypotension and bradycardia occur due to sympathetic tone loss. Respiratory function compromise occurs if the intercostal or abdominal muscles are involved.
3. The 'reflex' or chronic phase ensues, whereby changes in the spinal cord lead to the return of sympathetic output from the cord along with hypertonia and exaggerated reflexes. During this phase, autonomic reflexia is of prime concern to the anaesthetist.

Autonomic Dysreflexia

In patients with a spinal cord injury at T6 or above, the presence of a continuous noxious stimulus below the level of the injury may cause an exaggerated response of the sympathetic nervous system. This is called autonomic dysreflexia. It occurs after the initial spinal shock phase of a spinal cord injury but may occur days or weeks later, and patients differ in their sensitivity to any given stimulus to provoke a response.

The commonest stimuli which cause autonomic dysreflexia include distended bladder, distended rectum, and skin lesions including pressure sores, in growing toenails or superficial skin infections. Other stimuli include intra-abdominal pathology such as bowel obstruction, perforated peptic ulceration or acute appendicitis when autonomic dysreflexia may be the only sign of significant intra-abdominal pathology. Uterine contractions during pregnancy may also provoke autonomic dysreflexia.

Box 7.3   Symptoms of Autonomic Dysreflexia

Pounding headache
Sweating of the face, neck and shoulders
Flushing and blotching of the skin above the level of the cord lesion
Blurred vision or 'seeing spots'
Nasal congestion
Bradycardia
Hypertension
Anxiety
Tightness in the chest, chest pain, palpitations or shortness of breath

---

Any one of the signs and symptoms listed in Box 7.3 may indicate a dysreflexic attack.

The management of autonomic dysreflexia is initially directed towards sitting the patient up and recording the blood pressure every 3–5 minutes until symptoms subside, and identifying the cause. The patient should be examined for a distended bladder; in situ catheters may become blocked, kinked or twisted. Patients who usually practice intermittent catheterisation should be catheterised and patients who have an indwelling suprapubic catheter should be catheterised per urethra. If bladder drainage does not resolve symptoms, the patient's rectum should be emptied. The patient should remain as head-up as possible during these procedures. If symptoms persist and the blood pressure remains elevated and no easily treatable cause is identified, sublingual nifedipine 10 mg (as a broken capsule under the tongue) should be administered and the patient's blood pressure monitored for the next 2 hours. Treatment with nifedipine is contraindicated in patients with significant aortic stenosis, unstable or acute angina or within one month of having had a myocardial infarction.

Failure to achieve a satisfactory reduction in blood pressure carries a risk of stroke. If provoking stimuli cannot be identified, there must be a high index of suspicion of intra-abdominal sepsis. In this group of patients, peritonism does not cause abdominal pain and abdominal guarding is absent as there is no abdominal muscle innervation.

Other Cardiovascular Changes

There is tendency to orthostatic hypotension in the first few weeks after injury but gradual adaptation occurs, which is due to a rise in rennin levels. The gradual tolerance to the upright position is also due to cerebral autoregulation changes.

Respiratory Changes

Tetraplegic patients usually have a rapid, shallow breathing pattern due to paralysed thoracic musculature. They also have a reduced forced vital capacity which can be as low as 40% of predicted in the upright position. Paraplegics have an approximately 80% reduction. The forced expiratory volume in 1 second tends to be normal. The accessory muscles contribute up to 90% of ventilation in patients with no intercostal function. The loss of abdominal muscle function results in loss of active expiration, severely impaired cough and an expiratory reserve volume of close to zero. Retention of secretions and ventilation/perfusion mismatch occurs.

Bone

Significant osteoporosis predisposes these patients to fractures.

Temperature

A high spinal cord injury impairs the ability to shiver, vasodilate and sweat, and these patients are greatly affected by environmental temperature changes.

Skin

Pressure sores can occur early and decubitus ulcers have been reported as a result of 2 hours of pressure. The areas concerned are immobile, anaesthetic and have poor cutaneous circulatory control. Dependent areas become oedematous. Intravenous access can be difficult.

Blood

Patients exhibit a normochromic, normocytic anaemia and hypoalbuminaemia may be present. There is an increased risk of deep vein thrombosis.

Genito-urinary

Urinary tract infection, proteinuria, reflux and calculi occur commonly. Renal failure may rarely supervene.

Gastro-intestinal

Chronic spinal cord injured patients may have delayed gastric emptying. Acute abdominal signs are very difficult to interpret and an acute abdomen in the spinally injured patient may present with autonomic dysreflexia.

Drugs

Baclofen and tizanidine are the first-line treatments for spasticity. Baclofen has a relatively short plasma half-life but cerebrospinal levels are slower to change. Omitting one or two doses in the perioperative period is unlikely to have adverse effects, but complete cessation must be avoided due to the occurrence of rebound hyperspasticity. Dantrolene is the second line of treatment. Diazepam and clonazepam are used as adjuncts. Oxybutinin is used for bladder spasticity. Chronic pain is not uncommon and these patients are often on opiates. Many of them use cannabis.

Anaesthesia for Chronic Spasticity

If the patient has mild or infrequent spasms which do not interfere with the proposed surgery, does not have autonomic dysreflexia and the surgery does not involve handling viscera, then light sedation or no anaesthesia is an option. Infiltration anaesthesia or peripheral nerve blocks may be helpful where some sensation persists below the sensory level. Vasovagal attacks may occur.

Regional Anaesthesia

Regional anaesthesia can be used successfully. There is no evidence that spinal anaesthesia adversely affects or alters deficits in spinal cord injured patients, so it worth considering. It prevents autonomic dysreflexia, spasms and priapism. The level of the block is impossible to determine but loss of spasms helps to indicate that the block is working. Epidural analgesia is not as effective as spinal anaesthesia in preventing autonomic dysreflexia. However, many patients dislike regional anaesthesia and are fearful of losing what remaining sensation they have.

General Anaesthesia

General anaesthesia offers protection from spasms and autonomic dysreflexia but they can still occur and problems are lessened by increasing the depth of anaesthesia. Dramatic hypotension can occur on induction of anaesthesia. It may be necessary to ventilate patients with high spinal lesions solely due to pre-existing respiratory compromise, and ventilation may be required in the postoperative period following prolonged surgery. Careful attention to padding and positioning to prevent skin and pressure injuries is important. Warm the patient for all procedures, as body temperature falls rapidly and thermogenesis is limited.

In obstetrics, autonomic dysreflexia has been reported in labour. Other triggers are amniotomy, perineal distension, syntocinon usage, and vaginal instrumentation. Epidural analgesia is effective in preventing this complication. A urinary catheter will prevent bladder distension which is a triggering stimulus.

8

Spinal Surgery

Spinal surgery occurs on the entire spine from the cervical region to the sacrum. Often, surgery entails combined anterior and posterior approaches and operations are frequently prolonged in their nature.

Cervical Spine Surgery

Surgery of the cervical spine is usually performed for disc protrusion or spinal instability due to fractures, dislocations, sepsis, neoplasia or a variety of arthritic diseases, such as rheumatoid arthritis or ankylosing spondylosis. Significant proportions of patients are elderly and will have either concomitant systemic manifestations of their medical condition or other incidental diseases. They may be neurologically unstable (as in the patient with a cervical fracture) and, in addition, often have airway problems. The degenerative changes in the spine that occur with ageing are cervical spondylosis and spinal stenosis, which is often accompanied by a severe myelopathy or neuropathy. The main considerations of anaesthesia for cervical spine surgery are listed in Box 8.1.

Decompression and fusion procedures are performed either anteriorly or posteriorly or both. The problems of positioning the patients in the prone and supine positions are discussed in Chapter 1. Care needs to be taken when transferring the patients to the operating table and the anaesthetist should only take responsibility for ensuring that no untoward neck movements occur. The indications for the trans-oral approach are lesions occurring in the C1/C2 vertebrae leading to instability with the destruction of the axis. There may also be upward migration of the odontoid into the foramen magnum and with compression of the cord.

The most important task is first to assess the stability of the spine neurologically and, in such instances where there is a history of any abnormality of neurology, it is of the utmost importance to maintain the cervical spine in the neutral position. Patients with fractures often have their head immobilised by a halo traction. Intubation should proceed along the principles outlined in Box 3.1. Awake fibre-optic intubation is often the technique of choice when there are problems maintaining and

---

Box 8.1   Considerations for Cervical Spine Surgery

Reason for surgery
Pre-existing disease
Incidental disease
Neurological stability
Intubation techniques
Reinforced tracheal tube
Secure tracheal tube
Transfer of patients to operating table
Position for surgery – prone, supine
Consider spinal cord monitoring
Postoperative analgesia

---

securing the airway. Crico-thyroid puncture and a retrograde catheter intubation technique is also a helpful option in very difficult cases. Rheumatoid arthritis may lead to a limitation in mouth opening due to ankylosis of the temporo-mandibular joint and atlanto-axial instability may also occur.

Ongoing spinal cord monitoring should also be considered (see end of this chapter) in some cases. Postoperatively, all patients should be nursed in an HDU/ITU environment as postoperative haematoma with subsequent tracheal compression can occur. In prolonged cases, especially where the intubation and/or the surgery was difficult, it is advisable to leave the patient intubated and nursed in the head-up position until one is sure that all the swelling has subsided.

Thoracic Spinal Surgery

Thoracic spinal surgery encompasses a wide variety of procedures and approaches to the spine, ranging from simple discectomy and laminectomy to transthoracic resection and stabilisation of tumours and fractures. Primary or metastatic tumours can lead to vertebral instability and neurological changes, surgery therefore involves stabilisation and decompression of the cord to prevent neurological damage and, hopefully, to reverse any damage already done.

Surgery for spinal stenosis involves decompression of the cord by laminectomy plus decompression of the nerve roots by foraminotomy. The indications for fusion are existing or potential instability due to trauma, tumour, infection or degeneration. Patients with spondylolisthesis require fusion when the forward slip of one vertebra on another is greater than 50%. Patients with ankylosing spondylitis are particularly prone to fractures and may require correction of fixed flexion deformities of the spine by multiple segmental osteotomies. These procedures are particularly hazardous because of the potential for both intraoperative neurological catastrophe and massive blood loss.

When there are lesions at L1 and above, the diaphragm must be divided after the chest is opened. This involves all the complications of a thoracotomy. Access to lower lumbar segments may be provided via a retroperitoneal approach, and consequently a postoperative paralytic ileus is common. This can be exacerbated by opiate analgesia. The anaesthetic requirements for major thoraco-lumbar spinal surgery are shown in Box 8.2.

Whilst surgery often involves a thoracotomy, it is rare to need one-lung anaesthesia unless a thoracoscopic approach is used. The surgeon normally retracts the lung out of the surgical field. The anterior approach exposes the anterolateral portions of the vertebral bodies and is useful for exposing tumours and lesions involving an entire vertebral body as in infection or a crush fracture. This exposure also facilitates placement of graft and interbody fusion. Major haemorrhage during vertebral resection is common and anticipation of the timing of the major blood loss in these procedures is crucial.

Patients who have had a thoracotomy need ongoing measurement of the pulmonary function and patients having anterior surgery below the diaphragm should be monitored for the return of normal bowel sounds before resuming normal oral intake. Leakage of cerebrospinal fluid (CSF) is always a possibility and patients who have had radiotherapy are particularly vulnerable as these tissue planes become adherent to each other. Wherever possible, an epidural for both approaches affords considerable benefit for both the intraoperative management and postoperative pain relief. However, most major spinal procedures should have intraoperative spinal cord monitoring and it should be remembered that

---

Box 8.2   Anaesthetic Requirements for Thoraco-lumbar Surgery

Positioning – prone, anterior or lateral
Thoracotomy
Diaphragm involved in surgery
Hypotensive anaesthesia
Haemorrhage
Ability to monitor spinal cord function
Postoperative analgesia
HDU environment for haemodynamic and neurological monitoring

spinal evoked potentials, both sensory and motor, are markedly affected by local anaesthetics.

Lumbar Spine Surgery

The posterior approach is the most commonly used and optimum positioning, as always, is crucial. An ever increasing number of patients now undergo instrumentation in an effort to provide stronger fixation and fusion and, in the case of spinal injury, to facilitate earlier rehabilitation. The major features of anaesthesia are shown in Box 8.3.

There is an increased work of breathing in the prone position, so patients are electively ventilated. On a frame or Montreal mattress, it is important to ensure that the abdomen is free. If there is vena caval obstruction, the blood returns to the heart via the epidural veins and the surgical field suffers from venous congestion and an increased likelihood of haemorrhage. If the abdomen is free, normotension or mild hypotension is all that is necessary.

Sacrectomy

Sacrectomy is performed mainly for tumour excision and is performed either prone or by a combined posterior and anterior approach. Bowel and bladder resection by a general surgeon may be required with the fashioning of an ileal conduit and colostomy to facilitate access to the sacrum and because there will be complete destruction of all the sacral nerve roots. Haemorrhage can be catastrophic and coagulopathy can occur. Full invasive cardiovascular monitoring is necessary and the patients must be nursed in an ITU environment postoperatively. High lumbar or low thoracic epidural analgesia is very effective and can be used in the postoperative period.

The object of surgery, apart from the excision of the surgical lesion, is to preserve lower limb function. Partial sacrectomy may preserve bladder and bowel function. Occasionally, sacral nerve roots may be

---

Box 8.3   Anaesthetic Considerations for Lumbar Surgery

Position – prone or lateral
Eyes protected
Nerves protected
Tracheal tube secure
Frame to prevent vena cava compression
Need for hypotensive anaesthesia?
Postoperative analgesia

implanted after the tumour has been resected. This surgery is time consuming and its results are inconsistent, but it does offer the patient a chance of continence.

Operations on Coccyx
Coccygectomy is a common operation that is not especially debilitating for the patient. It is performed in the prone position and is not especially painful postoperatively.

Spinal Deformity (Scoliosis)
Patients with spinal deformity present at different ages for corrective spinal surgery. They range from mildly physiologically impaired adults to ventilator-dependent children with severe cardiac compromise. Scoliosis is defined as a lateral and rotational deformity of the spine. The classification of scoliosis is as shown in Box 8.4, and it is worth noting that most scoliosis is idiopathic, occurring at periods of maximum growth with a female preponderance. Early-onset idiopathic scoliosis has a profound effect on pulmonary function, especially if present before the age of 5 years. The congenital group consists of abnormalities of the vertebrae, spinal cord or both. Scoliosis is the most common curve but kyphosis, kyphoscoliosis and occasionally lordosis occur. It is

---

Box 8.4   Classification of Scoliosis Curve Patterns

Idiopathic
  Infantile, <4 years old
  Juvenile, 4–9 years
  Adolescent, 10 years to skeletal maturity
Congenital
  Deformity due to abnormal vertebrae
  Deformity due to abnormal spinal cord development
  Deformity due to mixed pathology
Neuromuscular
  Neuropathic causes, e.g. cerebral palsy
  Myopathic causes, e.g. muscular dystrophy
Associated with Neurofibromatosis
Mesenchymal
  Congenital
  Acquired
Trauma
  Vertebral
  Extravertebral, e.g. burn contracture
Irritational

estimated that 12% to 15% of this group have a cardiac abnormality and up to 20% have renal pathology.

Monitoring the severity and progression of a curve is performed by measuring the 'Cobb' angle. This is the angle subtended by the intersecting lines drawn perpendicular to the superior surface of the uppermost vertebrae and the inferior surface of the lowermost vertebrae of the major curve. The greater the angle, the more likely the progression to surgery. The degree of rotation may also be assessed by the movement of the pedicles towards the midline. Appreciation of rotation is important as it affects epidural placement of spinal cord monitoring electrodes and catheters.

It is important to understand the aims of the surgical procedure before assessing these patients. In a patient with juvenile scoliosis or an adolescent patient with an idiopathic curve, the goal may be:

• Prevention of disease progression;
• Maintenance of pulmonary function; or
• Limitation of pain.

This differs from other aetiologies such as neuropathic scoliosis secondary to cerebral palsy, where the aim is to maintain a stable posture and so facilitate seating in a wheelchair. This may help with general nursing and respiratory care.

A thoracotomy incision is used to provide anterior access to the spine and it may be part of a staged correction, in particular where there are large stiff thoracic curves or multiple curves. The diaphragm may be divided and the anterior longitudinal ligament resected, with excision of the anterior portions of the vertebral discs. This mobilises the vertebrae, aiding subsequent correction via a posterior approach. Some thoraco-lumbar curves may be fused and instrumented from the front.

The posterior approach provides exposure of the spine via a posterior longitudinal incision in the prone patient. The facet joints are excised and the vertebrae decorticated.

There are numerous instrumentation systems, all of which claim to distribute the force of distraction over the length of the fusion as opposed to older techniques that involved longitudinal distraction and laminar wiring. All of them are extremely expensive.

The decision to perform both procedures under the same anaesthetic or a week apart is never easy. Single-session surgery is usually reserved for patients who would be very difficult to manage postoperatively (i.e., severe special needs). It must be remembered that, even in ASA I patients, the combined approach is a severe physiological insult and the increased possibility of cord compromise must always be borne in mind.

Respiratory Compromise

Patients with spinal deformity are at risk of respiratory compromise. In extreme cases, this progresses to hypercapnic respiratory failure, pulmonary hypertension and death. Spirometry consistently demonstrates a restrictive pattern of lung volume reduction. Vertebral and rib cage abnormalities directly reduce lung and chest wall compliance. The deformity also reduces the force developed by respiratory musculature. There is increased ventilation–perfusion mismatching.

In all aetiologies of scoliosis, the lungs are developmentally abnormal. Alveolar and pulmonary vascular structure is abnormal and this may contribute to increased pulmonary vascular resistance. Estimation of the magnitude of respiratory impairment and its perioperative significance is an essential part of assessment of patients presenting for corrective spinal surgery.

A patient with good exercise tolerance and no clinical signs of respiratory distress is unlikely to provide a perioperative respiratory problem. However, additional factors that can contribute to postoperative respiratory morbidity can be sought. These include:

- A history of frequent respiratory tract infection;
- Poor nutritional status;
- Chronic aspiration and poor cough;
- Inability to cooperate with intervention such as physiotherapy; and
- Symptoms of nocturnal hypoventilation such as morning headache and daytime somnolence with frequent waking at night.

Such factors need to be considered as part of an overall picture but do add valuable information to aid planning of postoperative respiratory support. Assessment of FEV1 and FVC is mandatory in all cooperative patients. Predicted values are derived from arm span in patients who are unable to stand, or tibial length and values expressed as percentages of predicted values derived from published nomograms. It is not possible to dictate absolute values before which surgery is precluded or postoperative ventilation inevitable. Towards and below value of 30% of predicted, the possibility of postoperative respiratory failure increases. This is especially so if additional factors as described above are present. These cases may be extubated onto noninvasive ventilation (e.g. BiPAP) and this support is then weaned over a period of days. An anterior surgical approach is precluded in patients with severe respiratory compromise and recurrent chest infections, and the surgeon and anaesthetist need to be involved in these decisions. The patient must accept the possibility of (usually temporary) tracheostomy formation if they fail to manage on noninvasive support. A short period of elective invasive ventilation may be needed and these facilities must be available before starting anaesthesia.

Patients who are unable to cooperate in the performance of simple spirometry should have more specialised assessment, including sleep studies and echocardiography prior to surgery.

Deformity Assessment
Assessment of deformity also needs to be made. Thoracic curves, especially if greater than 100 degrees and associated with thoracic kyphosis, are most likely to be associated with pulmonary dysfunction. The effect on the respiratory system is greatest if the deformity has been present from infancy. Assessment of the aetiology of the deformity also aids evaluation. Myopathic conditions will have greater disruption of pulmonary function for equivalent curve angles. Patients with conditions such as cerebral palsy are at risk of aspiration and are unlikely to cooperate with some types of assessment and treatment. Such patients are at high risk of requiring postoperative respiratory support.

Pulmonary Assessment
Sleep studies describe monitoring of pulmonary function overnight. In its simplest form, this may be intermittent pulse oximetry. However, multichannel analysers are available, allowing assessment of transcutaneous carbon dioxide and oxygen tension as well as other indices, such as respiratory rate, oronasal airflow and even decibel meters for snoring assessment. Sleep studies are used to assess hypoventilation as indexed by hypoxaemia and hypercapnia. In neuromuscular disease, this first presents in rapid eye movement (REM) sleep before progressing to non-REM sleep and finally daytime occurrence. Daytime hypercapnia is unlikely if respiratory muscle strength is more than 30% of predicted and vital capacity more than 50% of predicted. Diurnal arterial blood gas analysis showing hypercapnia is thus strongly predictive of marked respiratory impairment. Significant night-time disordered breathing means the patient must be available for postoperative support. In myopathic scoliosis, this is also an indication that nocturnal noninvasive ventilation should be instituted. This should be started preoperatively to increase cooperation postoperatively. In Duchenne muscular dystrophy, scoliosis develops once the child has become wheelchair bound. In these boys, nocturnal noninvasive ventilation improves diurnal blood gas tensions and may

improve long-term survival. Once these patients develop significant diurnal hypercapnia, survival without nocturnal support may be as short as 10 months.

Cardiac Assessment

Echocardiography allows a noninvasive estimation of right ventricular function and pulmonary artery pressure. This investigation is useful in all patients with poor pulmonary function as indicated by blood gas tensions, spirometry, clinical condition or sleep studies.

Sixty per cent of patients with congenital vertebral anomalies demonstrate defects of other organ systems. Seven per cent of this group have cardiac abnormalities, the most common disorder being a ventricular septal defect. The incidence of congenital heart disease in idiopathic scoliosis is estimated at 3%. All patients require careful cardiac assessment. Any murmur should be assessed with echocardiography and a high index of suspicion much be maintained in cases of congenital scoliosis, where cardiac abnormality is relatively common.

Specific syndromes may be associated with cardiac pathology and clearly these cases need specific investigation. Boys with Duchenne muscular dystrophy have an intrinsic cardiomyopathy. Resting tachycardia may be the first sign of significant cardiac involvement. Echocardiography to assess cardiac impairment is mandatory in this group and all patients require a preoperative electrocardiogram.

Anaesthetic Management

Patients presenting for corrective spinal surgery present multiple problems. Anaesthetic assessment is difficult and often includes the specialised cardiac and respiratory investigations as discussed. It is time consuming but essential in order to plan perioperative care and give patients and family enough information to decide if they wish to embark on major surgery. The patient and family should be warned about the possibility of prolonged postoperative ventilation, tracheostomy and a negative outcome.

The anaesthetic management of these cases is difficult. The majority of cases with spinal deformity do not present an unusual airway challenge. However, certain patient groups may have skeletal stiffness or deformity that makes either airway maintenance or tracheal intubation difficult. This may be compounded by additional factors such as excess salivation or bulbar weakness. Patient's suffering from ankylosing spondylitis form an especially difficult group. The cervical spine may be fixed in a rigid kyphosis, mouth opening may be reduced and crico-arytenoid disease may occur.

The cervical spine is brittle and minimal trauma can produce fracture. In severe cases, tracheostomy formation is impossible due to head position. Clearly, a detailed plan for airway maintenance needs to be made and the patient informed of this plan in order to give necessary cooperation. Many techniques are available and the chosen method should depend on local skills, equipment and the severity and type of patient deformity. Succinylcholine is rarely used as a muscle relaxant to aid elective tracheal tube placement. Patients with muscular dystrophies seem to be at increased risk of rhabdomyolysis, independent of malignant hyperthermia following succinylcholine administration. Those with neuropathic and myopathic syndromes are at risk of an abnormal hyperkalaemic response to this drug. Many diseases have been associated with malignant hyperthermia (MH) but, in most cases, the relationship is unclear. Only central core disease is reported as strongly linked to MH. In other diseases, such as the myopathies, there is no definitive link.

Inhalation induction is common, particularly in the population of patients with special needs. Venous access and invasive monitoring are essential but may prove very time consuming and difficult to establish. Controlled hypotension to mean perfusion pressures of 50–60 mmHg facilitates surgery and definitely minimises blood loss. However, it must be remembered that, at continuous mean pressures of below 50 mmHg, there is a decrease in spinal cord blood flow. The introduction of the short-acting agent remifentanil combined with the judicious use of inhalational agents has made the intraoperative analgesia for this type of surgery considerably easier.

As with any major operation, sudden large volume intraoperative blood loss can occur any time and rapid response is essential. Epidural venous bleeding, once it starts, is very difficult to control and quick progression to finishing the instrumentation and closing the wound is called for. In all these patients, intraoperative spinal cord monitoring should be mandatory and is discussed at the end of the chapter.

Thoracic epidural analgesia sited preoperatively by the anaesthetist for the anterior approach or under direct vision intraoperatively during a posterior approach affords excellent postoperative analgesia. Where intraoperative spinal cord monitoring is not required, the epidural analgesia may be used throughout the procedure. Anecdotal evidence suggests that children and adults with special needs do better from a respiratory viewpoint and are easier to manage with effective epidural analgesia than those on opiate-based regimens.

All patients undergoing corrective spinal surgery should be nursed in a high dependency/intensive care area postoperatively, where their respiratory, haemodynamic and neurological status is assessed on an ongoing basis. In patients who have epidural analgesia running, strict protocols are required to respond to any change in neurology. It must be ascertained with certainty whether any neurological abnormality is due to the epidural or to the surgery itself. The epidural local anaesthetic infusion should be switched off and neurological recovery monitored. Alternative adequate analgesia must be given. If there is any element of doubt, the surgical team should be recalled to assess the need for any surgical intervention such as evacuation of a haematoma. Long-term intensive care stay is common in patients with special needs and in patients who have significant postoperative respiratory compromise and, as previously stated, these patients require attention to detail throughout what is often a protracted hospital stay.

Halo-tibial Traction

In severe scoliosis, halo-tibial traction provides a relatively safe and comfortable method of improving the preoperative correction of the deformity. It is particularly useful in staged surgical procedures to correct a rigid scoliosis and it is applied following the initial anterior release of soft tissues (congenital or infantile scoliosis).

The halo is applied whilst the child is still under anaesthetic in the supine position with the head and neck suspended over the end of the table. If the anaesthetist supports the head, accidental extubation is avoided. The halo is held to the head by four pins. Threaded pins are inserted from medial to lateral through the proximal tibia and stirrups are applied to each pin. Cords from each stirrup are yoked together and a weight of about 3 kg applied. An equal weight is also applied from the halo by a pulley.

The weights are increased daily to a maximum of one-third of body weight. Neurological function needs to be closely observed. Nursing care, which includes the avoidance of bed sores, is greatly facilitated by placing the child on a Stryker frame. This frame allows rotation of the child in the axis of the traction. The complications of halo-tibial traction are shown in Box 8.5.

The child presents for the second stage of surgery still on traction. Tracheal intubation may now be difficult and the surgeon must be present to provide assistance. Once surgery is completed, the halo and tibial pins can be removed.

Spinal Cord Monitoring

Major spinal procedures are associated with a small but very definite incidence of postoperative neurological morbidity. The devastating

---

Box 8.5   The Complications of Halo-tibial Traction

Infection of the pin sites leading to osteomeylitis
Skull penetration with extradural abscess formation
Cranial nerve palsies
Brachial plexus palsies
Paraplegia and tetraplegia
Cast syndrome

---

effect of postoperative paraplegia, particularly in a young previously fit patient, has made unmonitored major spinal surgery a thing of the past. The risk of spinal cord injury during major surgery has been quantified and is reported to range from 0.7–10%. Certain conditions are associated with an increased risk of neurological injury, including:

- Kyphosis;
- Severe scoliosis, especially that associated with neuromuscular disease;
- Spinal trauma where there is instability; or
- Previous neurological deficit.

Patients with spinal tumours are also vulnerable. Following surgery for repair of aortic aneurysm, which requires clamping of the aorta and hence interference with the blood supply of the distal spinal cord, the incidence of partial or complete paraplegia has been reported to be as high as high as 40%. Any operation where corrective forces are to be applied to the spine, the canal involved, or an osteotomy carried out in the immediate vicinity of the cord may warrant spinal cord monitoring.

Various tests have been used to monitor spinal cord function and include:

- Wake up testing;
- Somatosensory evoked potential monitoring;
- Motor evoked potential monitoring.

The wake up test was first described by Stagnara in 1973. This involves waking the patient after the first spinal correction has been carried out by the surgeon. The patient is instructed to move their limbs to demonstrate preservation of motor function. This may need to be repeated at intervals during surgery. Most anaesthetists are alarmed at the prospect of attempting to elicit a meaningful response from the awakening patient in the prone position with a tracheal tube in situ! This form of assessment is now discouraged. The complications of accidental extubation, line displacement, air embolus and dislodgement of spinal instrumentation make it unsafe.

The development of neurophysiological monitoring of the cord has depended on basic scientific observations of central nervous system activity evoked by stimulation of peripheral nerves. Monitoring these evoked potentials involves isolating a single low-amplitude response from a background of random cortical electrical activity to produce a standard wave form. Modern computer technology and microprocessor signal averaging techniques have allowed widespread use of this method of continuously monitoring the integrity of the spinal cord during surgery. Somatosensory evoked potential monitoring (SSEP) has been used for more than 20 years and the application of motor evoked potential (MEP) monitoring, although still being developed, is becoming more widespread. Sensory and motor pathways can be damaged separately during surgery but the problem of monitoring them simultaneously exists.

The measurement of SSEPs involves the stimulation of a peripheral nerve and the detection of the afferent signal further along the sensory pathway. The stimulating electrode is normally a standard electrocardiograph electrode. The recording electrode may be placed in the epidural space, over the spinal process of the second cervical vertebra or on the skin over the cerebral cortex. The site of the stimulus and recording must be appropriate to the site of the potential cord damage (i.e. stimulating electrodes are caudad and recording electrodes are cephalad to the operative field). The stimulus site must be appropriate for the site of potential cord damage. There is little benefit in stimulating the ulna nerve when surgery is being carried out on the lumbar spine. Epidural electrodes are sited intraoperatively during posterior lumbar surgery or percutaneously by the anaesthetist for anterior spinal surgery. Scalp electrodes are sited over the somatosensory cortex of the scalp.

Commonly used stimulating sites in the lower limb include the posterior tibial nerve at the ankle (almost exclusively the L_5 nerve root) and the sural nerve (almost exclusively S_1), the peroneal nerve below the head of the fibula at the knee and the tibial nerve in the popliteal fossa. In the upper limb, the median and ulna nerves can be stimulated at the wrist.

SSEPs are very stable irrespective of the general anaesthetic used. Epidurally administered local anaesthetics significantly reduce the amplitude of the recorded wave but not in a dose-related manner. They are best avoided until neurophysiological measurements are complete. SSEP stimulating electrodes at the wrist may interfere with the fixation of intravenous cannulae and the siting of arterial lines. Additionally, the SSEP stimulus may create artefacts in the electrocardiograph and the use of the diathermy causes artefacts in the SSEP recordings.

MEPs are very sensitive to thiopentone, nitrous oxide, halogenated volatile agents and muscle relaxants. Decreases in the amplitude of MEPs are probably an earlier indication of spinal cord injury rather than decreases in SSEP amplitude. MEPs are obtained by stimulating the motor cortex or spinal cord and recording from a peripheral nerve, or from the muscle in which an action potential has been generated by the peripheral nerve. As with SSEPs, the stimulating and recording electrodes must be placed according to the operating field and the site of potential cord damage but, in contrast to SSEPs, the stimulating electrodes are cephalad and the recording electrodes are caudad. An amplitude decrease of 50% is considered significant.

Cord perfusion is important in both spinal and vascular surgery. Normotension is vital if a decrease in SSEP or MEP occurs. Cord function should be monitored throughout the period of wound closure and into the recovery period. Postoperatively, monitoring takes the place of regular assessment of sensation and movement. Any deficit must be noted and the surgeon informed. An HDU environment is ideal for the first 24 hours after surgery.

9

Acute and Chronic Pain Relief

Postoperative analgesia and the management of chronic pain in orthopaedic patients will be discussed in this chapter.

Acute Postoperative Analgesia

Surgery on bone is painful because of the huge periosteal nerve supply. Many orthopaedic operations are accompanied by several days of enforced bed rest. Apart from the humanitarian and psychological advantages of good analgesia, it is important that pain does not inhibit the capacity of the patient to breath normally, cough well and take part in active physiotherapy, thereby reducing the chances of developing a chest infection. This is especially important for the elderly. As a rule, good analgesia makes for early mobilisation and better rehabilitation.

A general plan is necessary for all patients and this is shown in Box 9.1.

The importance of a preoperative visit and explanation of any postoperative procedures cannot be overemphasised. Consent for unusual routes of administration, especially rectal drugs, must be taken.

Systemic Drugs

Nonsteroidal anti-inflammatory drugs (NSAIDs), in isolation or in combination with paracetamol, codeine or dihydrocodeine, are often used and are good for bone pain, but one must remember their side effects:

- Gastric ulceration;
- Decreased platelet aggregation;
- Hypersensitivity;
- Renal impairment; and
- Their potential for drug interactions.

There is good evidence that the use of NSAIDs impairs the uniting of bone following fracture or osteotomy. Many spinal surgeons will not allow their patients to take NSAIDs following surgery for spinal fusion.

Box 9.1   General Plan of Postoperative Analgesia

Preoperative assessment and patient discussion
Premedication
Systemic drugs
Nonsteroidal anti-inflammatory drugs
Opiates
Route – oral, intramuscular, intravenous, subcutaneous, rectal
Mode of administration – patient controlled or nursing staff
Nature – continuous versus intermittent
Regional anaesthetic techniques
Local anaesthetic alone
Addition of opiate
Route – epidural, caudal, spinal, specific nerves, wound
Mode – at surgery, intermittent bolus, infusion
Miscellaneous techniques
Steroids
Entonox
Benefits versus side effects
Follow-up

This is particularly important in adults where spinal non-union carries a significant morbidity. Morphine is the most commonly used systemic drug and is still used occasionally on an intermittent intramuscular basis. For bigger orthopaedic procedures, morphine is commonly prescribed as an intravenous patient-controlled device. A 1 mg bolus with a 5-minute lockout and a 20 mg 4-hourly dosages usually suffices for most adult patients. Morphine makes patients confused, vomit, constipated, and is less than ideal, and other techniques should be sought in the elderly especially.

Regional Techniques

Local anaesthetic drugs, either alone or in combination with opiates such as diamorphine or fentanyl, are commonly used after surgery. The most common technique for ongoing postoperative analgesia in the lower limb and for pelvic surgery is epidural analgesia. A dosage of 1–15 ml of bupivacaine 0.1% with fentanyl 2 mg/ml suffices but the patient must be managed in a facility with suitably trained staff. Many hospitals now have peripatetic 'acute pain teams' who manage epidural analgesia on the general wards with efficacy and safety. All staff on wards where patients with ongoing regional techniques are nursed must be conversant with signs signifying the need for more expert input.

Nerve blocks provide suitable analgesia in a variety of settings:

- Femoral nerve block;
- Ankle block;
- Brachial plexus block;
- Interscalene block; and
- Ulnar, median and radial nerve blocks.

A 'single-shot' femoral nerve block is often used to stop quadriceps spasm after knee surgery. An ankle block is suitable for lessening systemic drug requirement after foot and toe surgery. An interscalene is suitable for shoulder and upper limb surgery, and can be extended as a postoperative infusion for analgesia. The patient must be warned of the inability to move the arm after such a block. Hand surgery pain relief can be provided by ulnar, median and radial nerve blocks and by local infiltration. It is important to monitor the function of any block because the anaesthetist will be partially held responsible if any nerve damage is found postoperatively in which a block has been inserted. It is also vital to inform the surgeon of the presence and possible duration of any nerve block that the anaesthetist has performed or plans to perform. If the proposed surgery is in an area where nerve damage is likely, many surgeons prefer to 'know the worst' as early as possible and also prefer that local anaesthetic techniques are avoided altogether.

Miscellaneous Methods
The most important of these is the use of entonox, which is used to assist in the removal of drains from painful sites or to carry out painful dressing changes.

Patients must be followed up to ensure that high-quality analgesia is provided. Remember, immobilising a broken bone can bring huge relief. Fractures and dislocations after reduction and splinting in plaster of Paris cast often require only modest analgesia postoperatively. Increasing pain and parasthesia is an indication to look for another cause, e.g. nerve entrapment or ischaemia to the limb.

Chronic Pain Relief
Many patients with orthopaedic and rheumatological complaints attend chronic pain clinics. The general principles of treatment are shown in Box 9.2.

These patients can easily be divided into two groups: those with non-malignant disease or malignant disease.

Box 9.2   Principles of Chronic Orthopaedic Pain Treatment

Multidisciplinary
Inpatient or outpatient
Benefits versus side effects
Systemic drug treatments
Regional analgesic techniques
Complementary therapy
Follow-up

Non-malignant Disease

Non-malignant pain is often managed in the out-patient chronic pain clinic and systemic drugs are often used. Opiates in the form of transdermal fentanyl or oral morphine sulphate are used in situations such as the patient with 'failed back surgery'. The benefits of analgesia must be tempered by the potential side effects of opiates. Regional analgesia is also often used, especially for chronic back pain. Epidural steroids often help with pain associated with nerve root compression. Facet joint blocks and dorsal root ganglion blockade is also used. Trigger point injections of local anaesthetic and steroids are also helpful. Complementary therapies are frequently used. Acupuncture and transcutaneous nerve stimulators help and have next to no side effects.

Malignant Disease

Malignant bone pain is difficult to treat. Patients need to be assessed carefully and are often admitted to as in-patients. Treatment is either palliative or curative. Management is multidisciplinary and involves surgeons and oncologists. Care of the terminally ill is becoming the remit of the Palliative Care Team which frequently has good expertise amongst its members. Consideration as to the quality of the patient's life is paramount. Many of these patients are young and wish for an active lifestyle. Again, treatment involves systemic drugs, regional blockade and complementary therapies, and the benefits must be balanced by the potential for side effects. Regular follow-up of patients is essential.

10

Nerve Blocks

Orthopaedic surgery lends itself to the use of regional nerve blockade more than any other branch of surgery. The use of a peripheral nerve stimulator is essential to improve the success of individual nerve blocks. Nerve blocks need to be demonstrated to the trainee and, in this chapter, we shall just deal with the main aspects of the most common blocks. The proposal to use any nerve blockade, and its possible complications, must be discussed with the patient, and this must be documented. Mark the side and site of the blockade at this time.

Eliciting muscle twitches with a nerve stimulator in a painful limb is inconsiderate and leads to poor patient cooperation and often to technique failure. Give adequate analgesia and/or sedation to these patients.

Remember, although the success rate of nerve blocks increases with practice, no anaesthetist achieves 100% success. If the block fails, consider:

- Abandoning surgery (only in extreme circumstances);
- A different nerve block (if applicable and nontoxic doses of local anaesthetic have been used); and
- General anaesthesia – there is no such thing as a 'failed general anaesthetic'.

It is also important to remember that diabetics and patients on steroids are particularly at risk from the infective complications of local nerve blockade. A single dose of prophylactic antibiotic is recommended when performing blocks in these groups of patients.

Drugs

Surprisingly large volumes (20–30 ml) are needed when blocking individual nerves. It is desirous to use long-acting drugs such as l-bupivacaine in a nontoxic dose (2 mg/kg/4 hours) to achieve a long-lasting effect. Catheter techniques are often used to provide analgesia for longer than 10 hours in the postoperative phase.

It is important to remember not to add adrenaline to the local anaesthetic when performing blocks near terminal arteries. The addition of 5 µg/ml of adrenaline prolongs the duration of some blocks by up to 3 hours.

Upper Limb Blocks

Upper limb blocks are usually performed in combination with general anaesthesia but can easily be used alone to provide analgesia for surgery. The brachial plexus can be blocked in many ways and individual nerves can be blocked distally quite easily.

Anatomy

The upper limb is supplied by the brachial plexus and this is formed from the primary anterior rami of C5–8 and T1. These emerge from the intervertebral foramina and form roots at the level of the scalene muscles, and trunks (C5–6 – upper, C7 – middle, C8, T1 – lower) in the lower part of the posterior triangle of the neck. Each trunk divides into divisions (anterior and posterior) behind the clavicle and the cords are formed at the outer border of the first rib where they enter the axilla in the proximity of the axillary artery. The branches arise from the cords and the individual nerves arise from the branches (radial [C5–8, T1], median [C5–8, T1], and ulnar [C7–8, T1]). It is worth remembering that the musculocutaneous (C5–7) and radial nerves exit the fascial sheath high in the axilla.

Brachial Plexus

There are many techniques of brachial plexus blockade. We only use two techniques:

• The interscalene; and
• The axillary.

Interscalene Technique

The technique of the interscalene block is to position the patient supine with the head turned to the opposite side on one pillow. A line is drawn from the cricoid cartilage that intersects the posterior border of the sternomastoid muscle. Scalenus anterior can be palpated under this muscle and by moving the fingers laterally the interscalene groove can be palpated. A needle is inserted perpendicularly and caudally until it 'pops' into the sheath. Shoulder movement should occur at 0.5 mÅ and then after aspiration up to 40 ml of local anaesthetic solution can be given. The complications of the block are shown in Box 10.1.

> **Box 10.1   Complications of Interscalene Brachial Plexus Block**
>
> Horner's syndrome if stellate ganglion involved (15%)
> Arterial puncture (common carotid artery)
> Venous puncture (internal jugular)
> Phrenic nerve block in all cases
> Recurrent laryngeal nerve palsy (10%)
> Intrathecal injection (rare)

Axillary Technique

The axillary approach is performed with the patient supine and the arm abducted with the elbow flexed. The axillary artery is palpated high in the axilla and a needle passes either above or below the artery until it 'clicks' into the fascial sheath. The main complication is inadvertent arterial injection and aspiration is essential prior to the injection of up to 40 ml of local anaesthetic. This approach is unsuitable for shoulder surgery.

Wrist Block

The median nerve can be blocked between the palmaris longus and the flexor carpi radialis tendons. As the needle passes through the flexor retinaculum, a resistance can be felt and up to 5 ml of local anaesthetic can be given. The ulnar nerve is blocked lateral to the tendon of flexor carpi ulnaris at a depth of 1 cm and up to 3 ml of local anaesthetic is needed. The radial nerve is entirely sensory and is blocked by means of subcutaneous infiltration over the posterior aspect of the wrist.

Digital Nerve Blocks

Nerves to the digits are blocked by injecting 3 ml of local anaesthetic on either side of the phalanx. Do not use adrenaline-containing solutions.

Epidural and Spinal Analgesia

Spinal and epidural analgesia are commonly used to provide anaesthesia and postoperative analgesia for surgery on the lower limbs and pelvis. Caudal, lumbar, and thoracic techniques are commonly used. Caudal analgesia is often used to provide analgesia in children. Patients with epidural infusions must be nursed in an appropriate environment. A high dependency unit is ideal as a one-to-one nurse to patient ratio exists. In this environment, any anaesthetic complications of the block can be observed for. It is important to differentiate them from surgical complications. This is especially true for spinal

---

Box 10.2   Considerations for Epidural Analgesia

Technique of insertion
Additional hypotension from surgical haemorrhage
Where to nurse patient
Complications of block
Hypotension
Accidental subarachnoid insertion
Accidental intravenous injection
Epidural haematoma
Masks surgical complications
Needle insertion nerve damage
Infection

---

surgery, as an epidural haematoma from surgical or anaesthetic causes will be masked by an epidural infusion. This, of course, would be catastrophic for the patient. The main considerations of epidural usage are shown in Box 10.2.

Both lumbar and thoracic epidurals can be sited with the patient awake but this is often impossible in patients with trauma, fractures and scoliosis and, as a rule, we favour the insertion of epidurals with the patient anaesthetised.

Epidurals are often used to assist the surgeon by minimising blood loss and improving the surgical field. Controlled hypotension by this means is useful but can be potentially fatal if sudden catastrophic surgical haemorrhage occurs. Haemorrhage in the hypotensive patient needs prompt resuscitation with fluids and vasopressors, and this fact cannot be overstated.

Infection, especially after spinal surgery, is always a possibility and, if an epidural catheter is also inserted, there is a greater risk of abscess formation or even meningitis. A high level of suspicion should exist. It is worth emphasising that all of these procedures require attention to a meticulous aseptic technique, including mask, cloves and a surgical gown.

Lower Limb Blocks

Lower limb blocks are commonly performed in combination with general anaesthesia to provide intraoperative analgesia and to provide prolonged postoperative pain relief. This relief for joint arthroplasty can be as long as 12 hours, which is the period of most pain. These blocks are also useful as the sole technique when general or epidural/spinal anaesthesia is difficult or impossible, as in patients with ankylosing spondylitis.

If there is a risk of compartment syndrome developing as a result of surgery, the use of blockade should be discussed with the surgeon as the block may mask the pain associated with the development of the syndrome.

Anatomy

Briefly, the nerve supply above the knee is from L2–4 (lumbar plexus) through the femoral, obturator and lateral cutaneous nerve of the thigh. Below the knee, it is L4–5 and S1–3. An extension of the femoral nerve can supply the medial cutaneous area of the calf and may extend as far as the first metatarso-phalangeal joint.

Most major hip surgery involves blocking of the lumbar plexus. The skin over a hip incision can be blocked by a lateral cutaneous nerve of the thigh block performed medial to the anterior superior iliac crest. Knee surgery involves blocking both the sciatic and lumbar plexus although a femoral nerve block in isolation is effective for postoperative pain in that it, especially, relieves quadriceps spasm.

Sciatic Nerve Plexus Block

This is not a common block and we prefer the posterior approach when used. The patient is placed in a lateral semi-prone position. The line between the greater trochanter and the posterior superior iliac crest is bisected and the perpendicular caudal line from this point at 5 cm is penetrated by a nerve-locating needle. The objective is to aim for gastrocnemius function at 0.5 mÅ. The local anaesthetic is then injected. Blockade is slow and can take up to 30 minutes. Permanent sciatic nerve damage has been reported from direct sciatic nerve injection.

Femoral '3 in 1' Blockade

This nerve is located lateral to the femoral artery at a level just below the inguinal ligament. The nerve is felt to 'pop' as it passes through the two fascial planes. Aim for gastrocnemius function at 0.5 mA, aspirate to ensure that the needle is not arterial and then inject the local anaesthetic. Digital pressure below the injection causes a rostral spread and blocks the femoral, lateral femoral cutaneous nerve and the obturator nerve – the '3 in 1' block.

Lumbar Plexus

The lumbar plexus is normally blocked at the L4–5 level with the patient in the lateral decubitus position. The needle is passed 3 cm caudal and 5 cm lateral to L4 and is passed onto the transverse process, and is then walked off this bony landmark. Aim for quadriceps function at

0.5 mÅ and then inject the local anaesthetic. There is a risk of epidural spread and renal damage with this block.

Ankle Block

Anaesthesia of the foot is performed to ensure analgesia of the foot. The deep and superficial peroneal nerves, the tibial nerve and the sural nerves need to be blocked. The sural nerve is blocked by infiltrating 5 ml of local anaesthetic subcutaneously lateral to the tendo-Achilles until the lateral malleolus is reached. The tibial nerve is lateral to the posterior tibial artery and infiltration here of 6 ml of local anaesthetic is effective. The deep peroneal nerve is located lateral to the dorsalis pedis artery and 3 ml infiltration is effective. The superficial peroneal nerves are blocked by a subcutaneous infiltration of local anaesthetic medially and laterally over the anterior aspect of the foot at the level of the palpation of the tibialis anterior artery palpation.

A saphenous nerve block is often also needed. It is blocked at the level of the tibial tuberosity and a subcutaneous injection from the tibial tuberosity to the medial tibial condyle is needed. Ten ml of local anaesthetic is required.

Index